My Period Tracker

A Super Simple Way to Track Your Menstruation for 5 Years

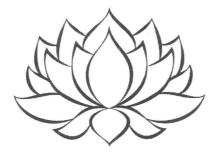

The Gathering Womb Wisdom

How to Use This Book

This book was designed to make tracking your period easy!

Each month has two pages to fill out. On the first page, start with the calendar and circle the days you are on your period.

SUN	MON	TUE	WED	THU	FRI	SAT
		1	2	3	4	5
6	7	8	9	10	11	12
13	14	(15)	(16)	(17)	(18)	(19)
(20)	21	22	23	24	25	26
27	28	29	30			

Check the boxes and fill in the spaces with your answers for when your period started and ended, the day length, and when the next one is expected.

Next, describe your flow and pain level for each day while on your period. Mark if your period was on time and if it feels normal or not.

FLOW	1	2	3	4	5	6
Spotting	☐	☐	☐	☐	☐	✗
Light	☐	☐	☐	☐	✗	☐
Medium	☐	☐	☐	✗	☐	☐
Heavy	✗	☐	✗	☐	☐	☐
Ultra	☐	✗	☐	☐	☐	☐
PAIN 1	☐	☐	☐	☐	✗	☐
2	☐	☐	☐	☐	☐	☐
3	☐	☐	✗	✗	☐	☐
4	✗	✗	☐	☐	☐	☐
5	☐	☐	☐	☐	☐	☐

The second page is where you record all of your period symptoms, from discomforts to cravings to emotions.

There is a Body Check section where you can keep track of your weight, exercise, and diet. This is also where your birth control, sexual activity, and any problems can be tracked.

Finally, use the annual charts to track the shifts in your period.

	1	2	3	4	5	6	7	8	9	10	11	12	13	14	15	16	17	18
Jan							x	x	x	x	x	x	x					
Feb								x	x	x	x	x	x	x	x			
Mar							x	x	x	x	x	x	x					
Apr								x	x	x	x	x	x	x				

My Period *Month:*_____ *Year:*_____

Start	SUN	MON	TUE	WED	THU	FRI	SAT

End

Day Length

Next Period Expected

Arrived:

☐ On Time ☐ Early ☐ Late

Feels:

☐ Normal ☐ See Doc

FLOW	1	2	3	4	5	6	7	8	9	10
Spotting	☐	☐	☐	☐	☐	☐	☐	☐	☐	☐
Light	☐	☐	☐	☐	☐	☐	☐	☐	☐	☐
Medium	☐	☐	☐	☐	☐	☐	☐	☐	☐	☐
Heavy	☐	☐	☐	☐	☐	☐	☐	☐	☐	☐
Ultra	☐	☐	☐	☐	☐	☐	☐	☐	☐	☐
PAIN 1	☐	☐	☐	☐	☐	☐	☐	☐	☐	☐
2	☐	☐	☐	☐	☐	☐	☐	☐	☐	☐
3	☐	☐	☐	☐	☐	☐	☐	☐	☐	☐
4	☐	☐	☐	☐	☐	☐	☐	☐	☐	☐
5	☐	☐	☐	☐	☐	☐	☐	☐	☐	☐

Period Symptoms

Discomfort: ☐ Cramps ☐ Mood Swings ☐ Headache ☐ Hunger
☐ Tender Breasts ☐ Back Pain ☐ Fatigue ☐ Acne ☐ Sleep Issues

Digestion: ☐ Nausea ☐ Ache ☐ Bloat ☐ Diarrhea ☐ Constipation

Cravings: ☐ Sweet ☐ Spice ☐ Salt ☐ Carb ☐ Cheese ☐ Alcohol

Emotions: ☐ Happy ☐ Energetic ☐ Motivated ☐ Calm ☐ Angry
☐ Irritated ☐ Sad ☐ Stressed ☐ Anxious ☐ Excited ☐ In Love

Body Check   *Weight:* _____

Exercise: ☐ Stretches ☐ Yoga ☐ Cardio ☐ Weights ☐ Impact

Diet: ☐ Healthy Eating ☐ Standard Diet ☐ Processed Food

Discharge Normal Colors: ☐ Clear ☐ White ☐ Pink ☐ Brown
   NOT Normal: ☐ Yellow ☐ Green ☐ Gray ☐ White Lumps

Problems: ☐ Itchy ☐ Burning ☐ Soreness ☐ Weird Discharge
☐ Funky Smell ☐ Odd Changes ☐ Pain with Peeing ☐ Pain with Sex

Sex: ☐ Nope ☐ Solo ☐ Girls Only ☐ Protected ☐ Unprotected

Birth Control: ☐ Condom ☐ IUD ☐ Pill ☐ Patch ☐ Implant
☐ Shot ☐ Vaginal Ring ☐ Tubal Ligation ☐ Partner Vasectomy

Notes

_____

_____

_____

_____

_____

_____

My Period *Month:_____ Year:_____*

	SUN	MON	TUE	WED	THU	FRI	SAT
Start							
End							
Day Length							
Next Period Expected							

Arrived:

☐ On Time ☐ Early ☐ Late

Feels:

☐ Normal ☐ See Doc

FLOW	1	2	3	4	5	6	7	8	9	10
Spotting	☐	☐	☐	☐	☐	☐	☐	☐	☐	☐
Light	☐	☐	☐	☐	☐	☐	☐	☐	☐	☐
Medium	☐	☐	☐	☐	☐	☐	☐	☐	☐	☐
Heavy	☐	☐	☐	☐	☐	☐	☐	☐	☐	☐
Ultra	☐	☐	☐	☐	☐	☐	☐	☐	☐	☐
PAIN 1	☐	☐	☐	☐	☐	☐	☐	☐	☐	☐
2	☐	☐	☐	☐	☐	☐	☐	☐	☐	☐
3	☐	☐	☐	☐	☐	☐	☐	☐	☐	☐
4	☐	☐	☐	☐	☐	☐	☐	☐	☐	☐
5	☐	☐	☐	☐	☐	☐	☐	☐	☐	☐

Period Symptoms

Discomfort: ☐ Cramps ☐ Mood Swings ☐ Headache ☐ Hunger
☐ Tender Breasts ☐ Back Pain ☐ Fatigue ☐ Acne ☐ Sleep Issues

Digestion: ☐ Nausea ☐ Ache ☐ Bloat ☐ Diarrhea ☐ Constipation

Cravings: ☐ Sweet ☐ Spice ☐ Salt ☐ Carb ☐ Cheese ☐ Alcohol

Emotions: ☐ Happy ☐ Energetic ☐ Motivated ☐ Calm ☐ Angry
☐ Irritated ☐ Sad ☐ Stressed ☐ Anxious ☐ Excited ☐ In Love

Body Check   *Weight:* _____

Exercise: ☐ Stretches ☐ Yoga ☐ Cardio ☐ Weights ☐ Impact

Diet: ☐ Healthy Eating ☐ Standard Diet ☐ Processed Food

Discharge Normal Colors: ☐ Clear ☐ White ☐ Pink ☐ Brown
    NOT Normal: ☐ Yellow ☐ Green ☐ Gray ☐ White Lumps

Problems: ☐ Itchy ☐ Burning ☐ Soreness ☐ Weird Discharge
☐ Funky Smell ☐ Odd Changes ☐ Pain with Peeing ☐ Pain with Sex

Sex: ☐ Nope ☐ Solo ☐ Girls Only ☐ Protected ☐ Unprotected

Birth Control: ☐ Condom ☐ IUD ☐ Pill ☐ Patch ☐ Implant
☐ Shot ☐ Vaginal Ring ☐ Tubal Ligation ☐ Partner Vasectomy

Notes

_____

_____

_____

_____

_____

_____

My Period *Month:*_____ *Year:*_____

Start	SUN	MON	TUE	WED	THU	FRI	SAT
End							
Day Length							
Next Period Expected							

Arrived:

☐ On Time ☐ Early ☐ Late

Feels:

☐ Normal ☐ See Doc

FLOW	1	2	3	4	5	6	7	8	9	10
Spotting	☐	☐	☐	☐	☐	☐	☐	☐	☐	☐
Light	☐	☐	☐	☐	☐	☐	☐	☐	☐	☐
Medium	☐	☐	☐	☐	☐	☐	☐	☐	☐	☐
Heavy	☐	☐	☐	☐	☐	☐	☐	☐	☐	☐
Ultra	☐	☐	☐	☐	☐	☐	☐	☐	☐	☐
PAIN 1	☐	☐	☐	☐	☐	☐	☐	☐	☐	☐
2	☐	☐	☐	☐	☐	☐	☐	☐	☐	☐
3	☐	☐	☐	☐	☐	☐	☐	☐	☐	☐
4	☐	☐	☐	☐	☐	☐	☐	☐	☐	☐
5	☐	☐	☐	☐	☐	☐	☐	☐	☐	☐

Period Symptoms

Discomfort: ☐ Cramps ☐ Mood Swings ☐ Headache ☐ Hunger
☐ Tender Breasts ☐ Back Pain ☐ Fatigue ☐ Acne ☐ Sleep Issues

Digestion: ☐ Nausea ☐ Ache ☐ Bloat ☐ Diarrhea ☐ Constipation

Cravings: ☐ Sweet ☐ Spice ☐ Salt ☐ Carb ☐ Cheese ☐ Alcohol

Emotions: ☐ Happy ☐ Energetic ☐ Motivated ☐ Calm ☐ Angry
☐ Irritated ☐ Sad ☐ Stressed ☐ Anxious ☐ Excited ☐ In Love

Body Check   *Weight:* _____

Exercise: ☐ Stretches ☐ Yoga ☐ Cardio ☐ Weights ☐ Impact

Diet: ☐ Healthy Eating ☐ Standard Diet ☐ Processed Food

Discharge Normal Colors: ☐ Clear ☐ White ☐ Pink ☐ Brown
NOT Normal: ☐ Yellow ☐ Green ☐ Gray ☐ White Lumps

Problems: ☐ Itchy ☐ Burning ☐ Soreness ☐ Weird Discharge
☐ Funky Smell ☐ Odd Changes ☐ Pain with Peeing ☐ Pain with Sex

Sex: ☐ Nope ☐ Solo ☐ Girls Only ☐ Protected ☐ Unprotected

Birth Control: ☐ Condom ☐ IUD ☐ Pill ☐ Patch ☐ Implant
☐ Shot ☐ Vaginal Ring ☐ Tubal Ligation ☐ Partner Vasectomy

Notes

_____

_____

_____

_____

_____

_____

My Period   *Month:*_____   *Year:*_____

Start	SUN	MON	TUE	WED	THU	FRI	SAT

End

Day Length

Next Period Expected

Arrived:

☐ On Time ☐ Early ☐ Late

Feels:

☐ Normal ☐ See Doc

FLOW	1	2	3	4	5	6	7	8	9	10
Spotting	☐	☐	☐	☐	☐	☐	☐	☐	☐	☐
Light	☐	☐	☐	☐	☐	☐	☐	☐	☐	☐
Medium	☐	☐	☐	☐	☐	☐	☐	☐	☐	☐
Heavy	☐	☐	☐	☐	☐	☐	☐	☐	☐	☐
Ultra	☐	☐	☐	☐	☐	☐	☐	☐	☐	☐
PAIN 1	☐	☐	☐	☐	☐	☐	☐	☐	☐	☐
2	☐	☐	☐	☐	☐	☐	☐	☐	☐	☐
3	☐	☐	☐	☐	☐	☐	☐	☐	☐	☐
4	☐	☐	☐	☐	☐	☐	☐	☐	☐	☐
5	☐	☐	☐	☐	☐	☐	☐	☐	☐	☐

Period Symptoms

Discomfort: ☐ Cramps ☐ Mood Swings ☐ Headache ☐ Hunger
☐ Tender Breasts ☐ Back Pain ☐ Fatigue ☐ Acne ☐ Sleep Issues

Digestion: ☐ Nausea ☐ Ache ☐ Bloat ☐ Diarrhea ☐ Constipation

Cravings: ☐ Sweet ☐ Spice ☐ Salt ☐ Carb ☐ Cheese ☐ Alcohol

Emotions: ☐ Happy ☐ Energetic ☐ Motivated ☐ Calm ☐ Angry
☐ Irritated ☐ Sad ☐ Stressed ☐ Anxious ☐ Excited ☐ In Love

Body Check   Weight: _____

Exercise: ☐ Stretches ☐ Yoga ☐ Cardio ☐ Weights ☐ Impact

Diet: ☐ Healthy Eating ☐ Standard Diet ☐ Processed Food

Discharge Normal Colors: ☐ Clear ☐ White ☐ Pink ☐ Brown
NOT Normal: ☐ Yellow ☐ Green ☐ Gray ☐ White Lumps

Problems: ☐ Itchy ☐ Burning ☐ Soreness ☐ Weird Discharge
☐ Funky Smell ☐ Odd Changes ☐ Pain with Peeing ☐ Pain with Sex

Sex: ☐ Nope ☐ Solo ☐ Girls Only ☐ Protected ☐ Unprotected

Birth Control: ☐ Condom ☐ IUD ☐ Pill ☐ Patch ☐ Implant
☐ Shot ☐ Vaginal Ring ☐ Tubal Ligation ☐ Partner Vasectomy

Notes

_____

_____

_____

_____

_____

_____

My Period　　*Month:*_____　　*Year:*_____

| | *Start* | | | SUN | MON | TUE | WED | THU | FRI | SAT |

Start

[ ]

End

[ ]

Day Length

[ ]

Next Period Expected

[ ]

	SUN	MON	TUE	WED	THU	FRI	SAT

Arrived:

☐ On Time ☐ Early ☐ Late

Feels:

☐ Normal ☐ See Doc

FLOW	1	2	3	4	5	6	7	8	9	10
Spotting	☐	☐	☐	☐	☐	☐	☐	☐	☐	☐
Light	☐	☐	☐	☐	☐	☐	☐	☐	☐	☐
Medium	☐	☐	☐	☐	☐	☐	☐	☐	☐	☐
Heavy	☐	☐	☐	☐	☐	☐	☐	☐	☐	☐
Ultra	☐	☐	☐	☐	☐	☐	☐	☐	☐	☐
PAIN 1	☐	☐	☐	☐	☐	☐	☐	☐	☐	☐
2	☐	☐	☐	☐	☐	☐	☐	☐	☐	☐
3	☐	☐	☐	☐	☐	☐	☐	☐	☐	☐
4	☐	☐	☐	☐	☐	☐	☐	☐	☐	☐
5	☐	☐	☐	☐	☐	☐	☐	☐	☐	☐

Period Symptoms

Discomfort: ☐ Cramps ☐ Mood Swings ☐ Headache ☐ Hunger
☐ Tender Breasts ☐ Back Pain ☐ Fatigue ☐ Acne ☐ Sleep Issues

Digestion: ☐ Nausea ☐ Ache ☐ Bloat ☐ Diarrhea ☐ Constipation

Cravings: ☐ Sweet ☐ Spice ☐ Salt ☐ Carb ☐ Cheese ☐ Alcohol

Emotions: ☐ Happy ☐ Energetic ☐ Motivated ☐ Calm ☐ Angry
☐ Irritated ☐ Sad ☐ Stressed ☐ Anxious ☐ Excited ☐ In Love

Body Check   Weight: _____

Exercise: ☐ Stretches ☐ Yoga ☐ Cardio ☐ Weights ☐ Impact

Diet: ☐ Healthy Eating ☐ Standard Diet ☐ Processed Food

Discharge Normal Colors: ☐ Clear ☐ White ☐ Pink ☐ Brown
  NOT Normal: ☐ Yellow ☐ Green ☐ Gray ☐ White Lumps

Problems: ☐ Itchy ☐ Burning ☐ Soreness ☐ Weird Discharge
☐ Funky Smell ☐ Odd Changes ☐ Pain with Peeing ☐ Pain with Sex

Sex: ☐ Nope ☐ Solo ☐ Girls Only ☐ Protected ☐ Unprotected

Birth Control: ☐ Condom ☐ IUD ☐ Pill ☐ Patch ☐ Implant
☐ Shot ☐ Vaginal Ring ☐ Tubal Ligation ☐ Partner Vasectomy

Notes

_____

_____

_____

_____

_____

_____

My Period *Month:*_____ *Year:*_____

Start	SUN	MON	TUE	WED	THU	FRI	SAT

End

Day Length

Next Period Expected

Arrived:

☐ On Time ☐ Early ☐ Late

Feels:

☐ Normal ☐ See Doc

FLOW	1	2	3	4	5	6	7	8	9	10
Spotting	☐	☐	☐	☐	☐	☐	☐	☐	☐	☐
Light	☐	☐	☐	☐	☐	☐	☐	☐	☐	☐
Medium	☐	☐	☐	☐	☐	☐	☐	☐	☐	☐
Heavy	☐	☐	☐	☐	☐	☐	☐	☐	☐	☐
Ultra	☐	☐	☐	☐	☐	☐	☐	☐	☐	☐
PAIN 1	☐	☐	☐	☐	☐	☐	☐	☐	☐	☐
2	☐	☐	☐	☐	☐	☐	☐	☐	☐	☐
3	☐	☐	☐	☐	☐	☐	☐	☐	☐	☐
4	☐	☐	☐	☐	☐	☐	☐	☐	☐	☐
5	☐	☐	☐	☐	☐	☐	☐	☐	☐	☐

Period Symptoms

Discomfort: ☐ Cramps ☐ Mood Swings ☐ Headache ☐ Hunger
☐ Tender Breasts ☐ Back Pain ☐ Fatigue ☐ Acne ☐ Sleep Issues

Digestion: ☐ Nausea ☐ Ache ☐ Bloat ☐ Diarrhea ☐ Constipation

Cravings: ☐ Sweet ☐ Spice ☐ Salt ☐ Carb ☐ Cheese ☐ Alcohol

Emotions: ☐ Happy ☐ Energetic ☐ Motivated ☐ Calm ☐ Angry
☐ Irritated ☐ Sad ☐ Stressed ☐ Anxious ☐ Excited ☐ In Love

Body Check   *Weight:* _____

Exercise: ☐ Stretches ☐ Yoga ☐ Cardio ☐ Weights ☐ Impact

Diet: ☐ Healthy Eating ☐ Standard Diet ☐ Processed Food

Discharge Normal Colors: ☐ Clear ☐ White ☐ Pink ☐ Brown
   NOT Normal: ☐ Yellow ☐ Green ☐ Gray ☐ White Lumps

Problems: ☐ Itchy ☐ Burning ☐ Soreness ☐ Weird Discharge
☐ Funky Smell ☐ Odd Changes ☐ Pain with Peeing ☐ Pain with Sex

Sex: ☐ Nope ☐ Solo ☐ Girls Only ☐ Protected ☐ Unprotected

Birth Control: ☐ Condom ☐ IUD ☐ Pill ☐ Patch ☐ Implant
☐ Shot ☐ Vaginal Ring ☐ Tubal Ligation ☐ Partner Vasectomy

Notes

_____

_____

_____

_____

_____

_____

My Period   *Month:*_____   *Year:*_____

Start	*SUN*	*MON*	*TUE*	*WED*	*THU*	*FRI*	*SAT*
End							
Day Length							
Next Period Expected							

Arrived:

☐ On Time ☐ Early ☐ Late

Feels:

☐ Normal ☐ See Doc

FLOW	1	2	3	4	5	6	7	8	9	10
Spotting	☐	☐	☐	☐	☐	☐	☐	☐	☐	☐
Light	☐	☐	☐	☐	☐	☐	☐	☐	☐	☐
Medium	☐	☐	☐	☐	☐	☐	☐	☐	☐	☐
Heavy	☐	☐	☐	☐	☐	☐	☐	☐	☐	☐
Ultra	☐	☐	☐	☐	☐	☐	☐	☐	☐	☐
PAIN 1	☐	☐	☐	☐	☐	☐	☐	☐	☐	☐
2	☐	☐	☐	☐	☐	☐	☐	☐	☐	☐
3	☐	☐	☐	☐	☐	☐	☐	☐	☐	☐
4	☐	☐	☐	☐	☐	☐	☐	☐	☐	☐
5	☐	☐	☐	☐	☐	☐	☐	☐	☐	☐

Period Symptoms

Discomfort: ☐ Cramps ☐ Mood Swings ☐ Headache ☐ Hunger
☐ Tender Breasts ☐ Back Pain ☐ Fatigue ☐ Acne ☐ Sleep Issues

Digestion: ☐ Nausea ☐ Ache ☐ Bloat ☐ Diarrhea ☐ Constipation

Cravings: ☐ Sweet ☐ Spice ☐ Salt ☐ Carb ☐ Cheese ☐ Alcohol

Emotions: ☐ Happy ☐ Energetic ☐ Motivated ☐ Calm ☐ Angry
☐ Irritated ☐ Sad ☐ Stressed ☐ Anxious ☐ Excited ☐ In Love

Body Check   *Weight:* _____

Exercise: ☐ Stretches ☐ Yoga ☐ Cardio ☐ Weights ☐ Impact

Diet: ☐ Healthy Eating ☐ Standard Diet ☐ Processed Food

Discharge Normal Colors: ☐ Clear ☐ White ☐ Pink ☐ Brown
   NOT Normal: ☐ Yellow ☐ Green ☐ Gray ☐ White Lumps

Problems: ☐ Itchy ☐ Burning ☐ Soreness ☐ Weird Discharge
☐ Funky Smell ☐ Odd Changes ☐ Pain with Peeing ☐ Pain with Sex

Sex: ☐ Nope ☐ Solo ☐ Girls Only ☐ Protected ☐ Unprotected

Birth Control: ☐ Condom ☐ IUD ☐ Pill ☐ Patch ☐ Implant
☐ Shot ☐ Vaginal Ring ☐ Tubal Ligation ☐ Partner Vasectomy

Notes

_____

_____

_____

_____

_____

_____

My Period

Month:_____ **Year:**_____

Start

	SUN	MON	TUE	WED	THU	FRI	SAT

End

Day Length

Next Period Expected

Arrived:

☐ On Time ☐ Early ☐ Late

Feels:

☐ Normal ☐ See Doc

FLOW	1	2	3	4	5	6	7	8	9	10
Spotting	☐	☐	☐	☐	☐	☐	☐	☐	☐	☐
Light	☐	☐	☐	☐	☐	☐	☐	☐	☐	☐
Medium	☐	☐	☐	☐	☐	☐	☐	☐	☐	☐
Heavy	☐	☐	☐	☐	☐	☐	☐	☐	☐	☐
Ultra	☐	☐	☐	☐	☐	☐	☐	☐	☐	☐
PAIN 1	☐	☐	☐	☐	☐	☐	☐	☐	☐	☐
2	☐	☐	☐	☐	☐	☐	☐	☐	☐	☐
3	☐	☐	☐	☐	☐	☐	☐	☐	☐	☐
4	☐	☐	☐	☐	☐	☐	☐	☐	☐	☐
5	☐	☐	☐	☐	☐	☐	☐	☐	☐	☐

Period Symptoms

Discomfort: ☐ Cramps ☐ Mood Swings ☐ Headache ☐ Hunger
☐ Tender Breasts ☐ Back Pain ☐ Fatigue ☐ Acne ☐ Sleep Issues

Digestion: ☐ Nausea ☐ Ache ☐ Bloat ☐ Diarrhea ☐ Constipation

Cravings: ☐ Sweet ☐ Spice ☐ Salt ☐ Carb ☐ Cheese ☐ Alcohol

Emotions: ☐ Happy ☐ Energetic ☐ Motivated ☐ Calm ☐ Angry
☐ Irritated ☐ Sad ☐ Stressed ☐ Anxious ☐ Excited ☐ In Love

Body Check   Weight: _____

Exercise: ☐ Stretches ☐ Yoga ☐ Cardio ☐ Weights ☐ Impact

Diet: ☐ Healthy Eating ☐ Standard Diet ☐ Processed Food

Discharge Normal Colors: ☐ Clear ☐ White ☐ Pink ☐ Brown
   NOT Normal: ☐ Yellow ☐ Green ☐ Gray ☐ White Lumps

Problems: ☐ Itchy ☐ Burning ☐ Soreness ☐ Weird Discharge
☐ Funky Smell ☐ Odd Changes ☐ Pain with Peeing ☐ Pain with Sex

Sex: ☐ Nope ☐ Solo ☐ Girls Only ☐ Protected ☐ Unprotected

Birth Control: ☐ Condom ☐ IUD ☐ Pill ☐ Patch ☐ Implant
☐ Shot ☐ Vaginal Ring ☐ Tubal Ligation ☐ Partner Vasectomy

Notes

_____

_____

_____

_____

_____

_____

My Period   *Month:_____*   *Year:_____*

Start	SUN	MON	TUE	WED	THU	FRI	SAT
	☐	☐	☐	☐	☐	☐	☐
End	☐	☐	☐	☐	☐	☐	☐
	☐	☐	☐	☐	☐	☐	☐
Day Length	☐	☐	☐	☐	☐	☐	☐
	☐	☐	☐	☐	☐	☐	☐
Next Period Expected							

Arrived:

☐ On Time ☐ Early ☐ Late

Feels:

☐ Normal ☐ See Doc

FLOW	1	2	3	4	5	6	7	8	9	10
Spotting	☐	☐	☐	☐	☐	☐	☐	☐	☐	☐
Light	☐	☐	☐	☐	☐	☐	☐	☐	☐	☐
Medium	☐	☐	☐	☐	☐	☐	☐	☐	☐	☐
Heavy	☐	☐	☐	☐	☐	☐	☐	☐	☐	☐
Ultra	☐	☐	☐	☐	☐	☐	☐	☐	☐	☐
PAIN 1	☐	☐	☐	☐	☐	☐	☐	☐	☐	☐
2	☐	☐	☐	☐	☐	☐	☐	☐	☐	☐
3	☐	☐	☐	☐	☐	☐	☐	☐	☐	☐
4	☐	☐	☐	☐	☐	☐	☐	☐	☐	☐
5	☐	☐	☐	☐	☐	☐	☐	☐	☐	☐

Period Symptoms

Discomfort: ☐ Cramps ☐ Mood Swings ☐ Headache ☐ Hunger ☐ Tender Breasts ☐ Back Pain ☐ Fatigue ☐ Acne ☐ Sleep Issues

Digestion: ☐ Nausea ☐ Ache ☐ Bloat ☐ Diarrhea ☐ Constipation

Cravings: ☐ Sweet ☐ Spice ☐ Salt ☐ Carb ☐ Cheese ☐ Alcohol

Emotions: ☐ Happy ☐ Energetic ☐ Motivated ☐ Calm ☐ Angry ☐ Irritated ☐ Sad ☐ Stressed ☐ Anxious ☐ Excited ☐ In Love

Body Check   *Weight:* _____

Exercise: ☐ Stretches ☐ Yoga ☐ Cardio ☐ Weights ☐ Impact

Diet: ☐ Healthy Eating ☐ Standard Diet ☐ Processed Food

Discharge Normal Colors: ☐ Clear ☐ White ☐ Pink ☐ Brown
   NOT Normal: ☐ Yellow ☐ Green ☐ Gray ☐ White Lumps

Problems: ☐ Itchy ☐ Burning ☐ Soreness ☐ Weird Discharge ☐ Funky Smell ☐ Odd Changes ☐ Pain with Peeing ☐ Pain with Sex

Sex: ☐ Nope ☐ Solo ☐ Girls Only ☐ Protected ☐ Unprotected

Birth Control: ☐ Condom ☐ IUD ☐ Pill ☐ Patch ☐ Implant ☐ Shot ☐ Vaginal Ring ☐ Tubal Ligation ☐ Partner Vasectomy

Notes

_____

_____

_____

_____

_____

_____

My Period   *Month:_____*   *Year:_____*

Start	SUN	MON	TUE	WED	THU	FRI	SAT

End

Day Length

Next Period Expected

Arrived:

☐ On Time ☐ Early ☐ Late

Feels:

☐ Normal ☐ See Doc

FLOW	1	2	3	4	5	6	7	8	9	10
Spotting	☐	☐	☐	☐	☐	☐	☐	☐	☐	☐
Light	☐	☐	☐	☐	☐	☐	☐	☐	☐	☐
Medium	☐	☐	☐	☐	☐	☐	☐	☐	☐	☐
Heavy	☐	☐	☐	☐	☐	☐	☐	☐	☐	☐
Ultra	☐	☐	☐	☐	☐	☐	☐	☐	☐	☐
PAIN 1	☐	☐	☐	☐	☐	☐	☐	☐	☐	☐
2	☐	☐	☐	☐	☐	☐	☐	☐	☐	☐
3	☐	☐	☐	☐	☐	☐	☐	☐	☐	☐
4	☐	☐	☐	☐	☐	☐	☐	☐	☐	☐
5	☐	☐	☐	☐	☐	☐	☐	☐	☐	☐

Period Symptoms

Discomfort: ☐ Cramps ☐ Mood Swings ☐ Headache ☐ Hunger
☐ Tender Breasts ☐ Back Pain ☐ Fatigue ☐ Acne ☐ Sleep Issues

Digestion: ☐ Nausea ☐ Ache ☐ Bloat ☐ Diarrhea ☐ Constipation

Cravings: ☐ Sweet ☐ Spice ☐ Salt ☐ Carb ☐ Cheese ☐ Alcohol

Emotions: ☐ Happy ☐ Energetic ☐ Motivated ☐ Calm ☐ Angry
☐ Irritated ☐ Sad ☐ Stressed ☐ Anxious ☐ Excited ☐ In Love

Body Check   Weight: _____

Exercise: ☐ Stretches ☐ Yoga ☐ Cardio ☐ Weights ☐ Impact

Diet: ☐ Healthy Eating ☐ Standard Diet ☐ Processed Food

Discharge Normal Colors: ☐ Clear ☐ White ☐ Pink ☐ Brown
  NOT Normal: ☐ Yellow ☐ Green ☐ Gray ☐ White Lumps

Problems: ☐ Itchy ☐ Burning ☐ Soreness ☐ Weird Discharge
☐ Funky Smell ☐ Odd Changes ☐ Pain with Peeing ☐ Pain with Sex

Sex: ☐ Nope ☐ Solo ☐ Girls Only ☐ Protected ☐ Unprotected

Birth Control: ☐ Condom ☐ IUD ☐ Pill ☐ Patch ☐ Implant
☐ Shot ☐ Vaginal Ring ☐ Tubal Ligation ☐ Partner Vasectomy

Notes

_____

_____

_____

_____

_____

_____

My Period   *Month:_____   Year:_____*

Start	SUN	MON	TUE	WED	THU	FRI	SAT

End

Day Length

Next Period Expected

Arrived:

☐ On Time ☐ Early ☐ Late

Feels:

☐ Normal ☐ See Doc

FLOW	1	2	3	4	5	6	7	8	9	10
Spotting	☐	☐	☐	☐	☐	☐	☐	☐	☐	☐
Light	☐	☐	☐	☐	☐	☐	☐	☐	☐	☐
Medium	☐	☐	☐	☐	☐	☐	☐	☐	☐	☐
Heavy	☐	☐	☐	☐	☐	☐	☐	☐	☐	☐
Ultra	☐	☐	☐	☐	☐	☐	☐	☐	☐	☐
PAIN 1	☐	☐	☐	☐	☐	☐	☐	☐	☐	☐
2	☐	☐	☐	☐	☐	☐	☐	☐	☐	☐
3	☐	☐	☐	☐	☐	☐	☐	☐	☐	☐
4	☐	☐	☐	☐	☐	☐	☐	☐	☐	☐
5	☐	☐	☐	☐	☐	☐	☐	☐	☐	☐

Period Symptoms

Discomfort: ☐ Cramps ☐ Mood Swings ☐ Headache ☐ Hunger
☐ Tender Breasts ☐ Back Pain ☐ Fatigue ☐ Acne ☐ Sleep Issues

Digestion: ☐ Nausea ☐ Ache ☐ Bloat ☐ Diarrhea ☐ Constipation

Cravings: ☐ Sweet ☐ Spice ☐ Salt ☐ Carb ☐ Cheese ☐ Alcohol

Emotions: ☐ Happy ☐ Energetic ☐ Motivated ☐ Calm ☐ Angry
☐ Irritated ☐ Sad ☐ Stressed ☐ Anxious ☐ Excited ☐ In Love

Body Check   Weight: _____

Exercise: ☐ Stretches ☐ Yoga ☐ Cardio ☐ Weights ☐ Impact

Diet: ☐ Healthy Eating ☐ Standard Diet ☐ Processed Food

Discharge Normal Colors: ☐ Clear ☐ White ☐ Pink ☐ Brown
    NOT Normal: ☐ Yellow ☐ Green ☐ Gray ☐ White Lumps

Problems: ☐ Itchy ☐ Burning ☐ Soreness ☐ Weird Discharge
☐ Funky Smell ☐ Odd Changes ☐ Pain with Peeing ☐ Pain with Sex

Sex: ☐ Nope ☐ Solo ☐ Girls Only ☐ Protected ☐ Unprotected

Birth Control: ☐ Condom ☐ IUD ☐ Pill ☐ Patch ☐ Implant
☐ Shot ☐ Vaginal Ring ☐ Tubal Ligation ☐ Partner Vasectomy

Notes

_____

_____

_____

_____

_____

_____

My Period   *Month:_____*   *Year:_____*

Start	SUN	MON	TUE	WED	THU	FRI	SAT
End							
Day Length							
Next Period Expected							

Arrived:

☐ On Time ☐ Early ☐ Late

Feels:

☐ Normal ☐ See Doc

FLOW	1	2	3	4	5	6	7	8	9	10
Spotting	☐	☐	☐	☐	☐	☐	☐	☐	☐	☐
Light	☐	☐	☐	☐	☐	☐	☐	☐	☐	☐
Medium	☐	☐	☐	☐	☐	☐	☐	☐	☐	☐
Heavy	☐	☐	☐	☐	☐	☐	☐	☐	☐	☐
Ultra	☐	☐	☐	☐	☐	☐	☐	☐	☐	☐
PAIN 1	☐	☐	☐	☐	☐	☐	☐	☐	☐	☐
2	☐	☐	☐	☐	☐	☐	☐	☐	☐	☐
3	☐	☐	☐	☐	☐	☐	☐	☐	☐	☐
4	☐	☐	☐	☐	☐	☐	☐	☐	☐	☐
5	☐	☐	☐	☐	☐	☐	☐	☐	☐	☐

Period Symptoms

Discomfort: ☐ Cramps ☐ Mood Swings ☐ Headache ☐ Hunger
☐ Tender Breasts ☐ Back Pain ☐ Fatigue ☐ Acne ☐ Sleep Issues

Digestion: ☐ Nausea ☐ Ache ☐ Bloat ☐ Diarrhea ☐ Constipation

Cravings: ☐ Sweet ☐ Spice ☐ Salt ☐ Carb ☐ Cheese ☐ Alcohol

Emotions: ☐ Happy ☐ Energetic ☐ Motivated ☐ Calm ☐ Angry
☐ Irritated ☐ Sad ☐ Stressed ☐ Anxious ☐ Excited ☐ In Love

Body Check   Weight: _____

Exercise: ☐ Stretches ☐ Yoga ☐ Cardio ☐ Weights ☐ Impact

Diet: ☐ Healthy Eating ☐ Standard Diet ☐ Processed Food

Discharge Normal Colors: ☐ Clear ☐ White ☐ Pink ☐ Brown
  NOT Normal: ☐ Yellow ☐ Green ☐ Gray ☐ White Lumps

Problems: ☐ Itchy ☐ Burning ☐ Soreness ☐ Weird Discharge
☐ Funky Smell ☐ Odd Changes ☐ Pain with Peeing ☐ Pain with Sex

Sex: ☐ Nope ☐ Solo ☐ Girls Only ☐ Protected ☐ Unprotected

Birth Control: ☐ Condom ☐ IUD ☐ Pill ☐ Patch ☐ Implant
☐ Shot ☐ Vaginal Ring ☐ Tubal Ligation ☐ Partner Vasectomy

Notes

_____

_____

_____

_____

_____

_____

My Period   *Month:*_____   *Year:*_____

Start	SUN	MON	TUE	WED	THU	FRI	SAT
End							
Day Length							
Next Period Expected							

Arrived:

☐ On Time ☐ Early ☐ Late

Feels:

☐ Normal ☐ See Doc

FLOW	1	2	3	4	5	6	7	8	9	10
Spotting	☐	☐	☐	☐	☐	☐	☐	☐	☐	☐
Light	☐	☐	☐	☐	☐	☐	☐	☐	☐	☐
Medium	☐	☐	☐	☐	☐	☐	☐	☐	☐	☐
Heavy	☐	☐	☐	☐	☐	☐	☐	☐	☐	☐
Ultra	☐	☐	☐	☐	☐	☐	☐	☐	☐	☐
PAIN 1	☐	☐	☐	☐	☐	☐	☐	☐	☐	☐
2	☐	☐	☐	☐	☐	☐	☐	☐	☐	☐
3	☐	☐	☐	☐	☐	☐	☐	☐	☐	☐
4	☐	☐	☐	☐	☐	☐	☐	☐	☐	☐
5	☐	☐	☐	☐	☐	☐	☐	☐	☐	☐

Period Symptoms

Discomfort: ☐ Cramps ☐ Mood Swings ☐ Headache ☐ Hunger
☐ Tender Breasts ☐ Back Pain ☐ Fatigue ☐ Acne ☐ Sleep Issues

Digestion: ☐ Nausea ☐ Ache ☐ Bloat ☐ Diarrhea ☐ Constipation

Cravings: ☐ Sweet ☐ Spice ☐ Salt ☐ Carb ☐ Cheese ☐ Alcohol

Emotions: ☐ Happy ☐ Energetic ☐ Motivated ☐ Calm ☐ Angry
☐ Irritated ☐ Sad ☐ Stressed ☐ Anxious ☐ Excited ☐ In Love

Body Check   Weight: _____

Exercise: ☐ Stretches ☐ Yoga ☐ Cardio ☐ Weights ☐ Impact

Diet: ☐ Healthy Eating ☐ Standard Diet ☐ Processed Food

Discharge Normal Colors: ☐ Clear ☐ White ☐ Pink ☐ Brown
   NOT Normal: ☐ Yellow ☐ Green ☐ Gray ☐ White Lumps

Problems: ☐ Itchy ☐ Burning ☐ Soreness ☐ Weird Discharge
☐ Funky Smell ☐ Odd Changes ☐ Pain with Peeing ☐ Pain with Sex

Sex: ☐ Nope ☐ Solo ☐ Girls Only ☐ Protected ☐ Unprotected

Birth Control: ☐ Condom ☐ IUD ☐ Pill ☐ Patch ☐ Implant
☐ Shot ☐ Vaginal Ring ☐ Tubal Ligation ☐ Partner Vasectomy

Notes

_____

_____

_____

_____

_____

_____

My Period   *Month:_____*   *Year:_____*

	SUN	MON	TUE	WED	THU	FRI	SAT
Start							
End							
Day Length							
Next Period Expected							

Arrived:

☐ On Time ☐ Early ☐ Late

Feels:

☐ Normal ☐ See Doc

FLOW	1	2	3	4	5	6	7	8	9	10
Spotting	☐	☐	☐	☐	☐	☐	☐	☐	☐	☐
Light	☐	☐	☐	☐	☐	☐	☐	☐	☐	☐
Medium	☐	☐	☐	☐	☐	☐	☐	☐	☐	☐
Heavy	☐	☐	☐	☐	☐	☐	☐	☐	☐	☐
Ultra	☐	☐	☐	☐	☐	☐	☐	☐	☐	☐
PAIN 1	☐	☐	☐	☐	☐	☐	☐	☐	☐	☐
2	☐	☐	☐	☐	☐	☐	☐	☐	☐	☐
3	☐	☐	☐	☐	☐	☐	☐	☐	☐	☐
4	☐	☐	☐	☐	☐	☐	☐	☐	☐	☐
5	☐	☐	☐	☐	☐	☐	☐	☐	☐	☐

Period Symptoms

Discomfort: ☐ Cramps ☐ Mood Swings ☐ Headache ☐ Hunger
☐ Tender Breasts ☐ Back Pain ☐ Fatigue ☐ Acne ☐ Sleep Issues

Digestion: ☐ Nausea ☐ Ache ☐ Bloat ☐ Diarrhea ☐ Constipation

Cravings: ☐ Sweet ☐ Spice ☐ Salt ☐ Carb ☐ Cheese ☐ Alcohol

Emotions: ☐ Happy ☐ Energetic ☐ Motivated ☐ Calm ☐ Angry
☐ Irritated ☐ Sad ☐ Stressed ☐ Anxious ☐ Excited ☐ In Love

Body Check   *Weight:* _____

Exercise: ☐ Stretches ☐ Yoga ☐ Cardio ☐ Weights ☐ Impact

Diet: ☐ Healthy Eating ☐ Standard Diet ☐ Processed Food

Discharge Normal Colors: ☐ Clear ☐ White ☐ Pink ☐ Brown
    NOT Normal: ☐ Yellow ☐ Green ☐ Gray ☐ White Lumps

Problems: ☐ Itchy ☐ Burning ☐ Soreness ☐ Weird Discharge
☐ Funky Smell ☐ Odd Changes ☐ Pain with Peeing ☐ Pain with Sex

Sex: ☐ Nope ☐ Solo ☐ Girls Only ☐ Protected ☐ Unprotected

Birth Control: ☐ Condom ☐ IUD ☐ Pill ☐ Patch ☐ Implant
☐ Shot ☐ Vaginal Ring ☐ Tubal Ligation ☐ Partner Vasectomy

Notes

_____

_____

_____

_____

_____

_____

My Period   *Month:_____*   *Year:_____*

Start	SUN	MON	TUE	WED	THU	FRI	SAT

End							

Day Length							

Next Period Expected

Arrived:

☐ On Time ☐ Early ☐ Late

Feels:

☐ Normal ☐ See Doc

FLOW	1	2	3	4	5	6	7	8	9	10
Spotting	☐	☐	☐	☐	☐	☐	☐	☐	☐	☐
Light	☐	☐	☐	☐	☐	☐	☐	☐	☐	☐
Medium	☐	☐	☐	☐	☐	☐	☐	☐	☐	☐
Heavy	☐	☐	☐	☐	☐	☐	☐	☐	☐	☐
Ultra	☐	☐	☐	☐	☐	☐	☐	☐	☐	☐
PAIN 1	☐	☐	☐	☐	☐	☐	☐	☐	☐	☐
2	☐	☐	☐	☐	☐	☐	☐	☐	☐	☐
3	☐	☐	☐	☐	☐	☐	☐	☐	☐	☐
4	☐	☐	☐	☐	☐	☐	☐	☐	☐	☐
5	☐	☐	☐	☐	☐	☐	☐	☐	☐	☐

Period Symptoms

Discomfort: ☐ Cramps ☐ Mood Swings ☐ Headache ☐ Hunger
☐ Tender Breasts ☐ Back Pain ☐ Fatigue ☐ Acne ☐ Sleep Issues

Digestion: ☐ Nausea ☐ Ache ☐ Bloat ☐ Diarrhea ☐ Constipation

Cravings: ☐ Sweet ☐ Spice ☐ Salt ☐ Carb ☐ Cheese ☐ Alcohol

Emotions: ☐ Happy ☐ Energetic ☐ Motivated ☐ Calm ☐ Angry
☐ Irritated ☐ Sad ☐ Stressed ☐ Anxious ☐ Excited ☐ In Love

Body Check   *Weight:* _____

Exercise: ☐ Stretches ☐ Yoga ☐ Cardio ☐ Weights ☐ Impact

Diet: ☐ Healthy Eating ☐ Standard Diet ☐ Processed Food

Discharge Normal Colors: ☐ Clear ☐ White ☐ Pink ☐ Brown
   NOT Normal: ☐ Yellow ☐ Green ☐ Gray ☐ White Lumps

Problems: ☐ Itchy ☐ Burning ☐ Soreness ☐ Weird Discharge
☐ Funky Smell ☐ Odd Changes ☐ Pain with Peeing ☐ Pain with Sex

Sex: ☐ Nope ☐ Solo ☐ Girls Only ☐ Protected ☐ Unprotected

Birth Control: ☐ Condom ☐ IUD ☐ Pill ☐ Patch ☐ Implant
☐ Shot ☐ Vaginal Ring ☐ Tubal Ligation ☐ Partner Vasectomy

Notes

_____

_____

_____

_____

_____

_____

My Period   *Month:_____*   *Year:_____*

Start	SUN	MON	TUE	WED	THU	FRI	SAT
End							
Day Length							
Next Period Expected							

Arrived:

☐ On Time ☐ Early ☐ Late

Feels:

☐ Normal ☐ See Doc

FLOW	1	2	3	4	5	6	7	8	9	10
Spotting	☐	☐	☐	☐	☐	☐	☐	☐	☐	☐
Light	☐	☐	☐	☐	☐	☐	☐	☐	☐	☐
Medium	☐	☐	☐	☐	☐	☐	☐	☐	☐	☐
Heavy	☐	☐	☐	☐	☐	☐	☐	☐	☐	☐
Ultra	☐	☐	☐	☐	☐	☐	☐	☐	☐	☐
PAIN 1	☐	☐	☐	☐	☐	☐	☐	☐	☐	☐
2	☐	☐	☐	☐	☐	☐	☐	☐	☐	☐
3	☐	☐	☐	☐	☐	☐	☐	☐	☐	☐
4	☐	☐	☐	☐	☐	☐	☐	☐	☐	☐
5	☐	☐	☐	☐	☐	☐	☐	☐	☐	☐

Period Symptoms

Discomfort: ☐ Cramps ☐ Mood Swings ☐ Headache ☐ Hunger
☐ Tender Breasts ☐ Back Pain ☐ Fatigue ☐ Acne ☐ Sleep Issues

Digestion: ☐ Nausea ☐ Ache ☐ Bloat ☐ Diarrhea ☐ Constipation

Cravings: ☐ Sweet ☐ Spice ☐ Salt ☐ Carb ☐ Cheese ☐ Alcohol

Emotions: ☐ Happy ☐ Energetic ☐ Motivated ☐ Calm ☐ Angry
☐ Irritated ☐ Sad ☐ Stressed ☐ Anxious ☐ Excited ☐ In Love

Body Check   Weight: _____

Exercise: ☐ Stretches ☐ Yoga ☐ Cardio ☐ Weights ☐ Impact

Diet: ☐ Healthy Eating ☐ Standard Diet ☐ Processed Food

Discharge Normal Colors: ☐ Clear ☐ White ☐ Pink ☐ Brown
  NOT Normal: ☐ Yellow ☐ Green ☐ Gray ☐ White Lumps

Problems: ☐ Itchy ☐ Burning ☐ Soreness ☐ Weird Discharge
☐ Funky Smell ☐ Odd Changes ☐ Pain with Peeing ☐ Pain with Sex

Sex: ☐ Nope ☐ Solo ☐ Girls Only ☐ Protected ☐ Unprotected

Birth Control: ☐ Condom ☐ IUD ☐ Pill ☐ Patch ☐ Implant
☐ Shot ☐ Vaginal Ring ☐ Tubal Ligation ☐ Partner Vasectomy

Notes

_____

_____

_____

_____

_____

_____

My Period   *Month:*_____   *Year:*_____

Start	SUN	MON	TUE	WED	THU	FRI	SAT
End							
Day Length							
Next Period Expected							

Arrived:

☐ On Time ☐ Early ☐ Late

Feels:

☐ Normal ☐ See Doc

FLOW	1	2	3	4	5	6	7	8	9	10
Spotting	☐	☐	☐	☐	☐	☐	☐	☐	☐	☐
Light	☐	☐	☐	☐	☐	☐	☐	☐	☐	☐
Medium	☐	☐	☐	☐	☐	☐	☐	☐	☐	☐
Heavy	☐	☐	☐	☐	☐	☐	☐	☐	☐	☐
Ultra	☐	☐	☐	☐	☐	☐	☐	☐	☐	☐
PAIN 1	☐	☐	☐	☐	☐	☐	☐	☐	☐	☐
2	☐	☐	☐	☐	☐	☐	☐	☐	☐	☐
3	☐	☐	☐	☐	☐	☐	☐	☐	☐	☐
4	☐	☐	☐	☐	☐	☐	☐	☐	☐	☐
5	☐	☐	☐	☐	☐	☐	☐	☐	☐	☐

Period Symptoms

Discomfort: ☐ Cramps ☐ Mood Swings ☐ Headache ☐ Hunger
☐ Tender Breasts ☐ Back Pain ☐ Fatigue ☐ Acne ☐ Sleep Issues

Digestion: ☐ Nausea ☐ Ache ☐ Bloat ☐ Diarrhea ☐ Constipation

Cravings: ☐ Sweet ☐ Spice ☐ Salt ☐ Carb ☐ Cheese ☐ Alcohol

Emotions: ☐ Happy ☐ Energetic ☐ Motivated ☐ Calm ☐ Angry
☐ Irritated ☐ Sad ☐ Stressed ☐ Anxious ☐ Excited ☐ In Love

Body Check   *Weight:* _____

Exercise: ☐ Stretches ☐ Yoga ☐ Cardio ☐ Weights ☐ Impact

Diet: ☐ Healthy Eating ☐ Standard Diet ☐ Processed Food

Discharge Normal Colors: ☐ Clear ☐ White ☐ Pink ☐ Brown
  NOT Normal: ☐ Yellow ☐ Green ☐ Gray ☐ White Lumps

Problems: ☐ Itchy ☐ Burning ☐ Soreness ☐ Weird Discharge
☐ Funky Smell ☐ Odd Changes ☐ Pain with Peeing ☐ Pain with Sex

Sex: ☐ Nope ☐ Solo ☐ Girls Only ☐ Protected ☐ Unprotected

Birth Control: ☐ Condom ☐ IUD ☐ Pill ☐ Patch ☐ Implant
☐ Shot ☐ Vaginal Ring ☐ Tubal Ligation ☐ Partner Vasectomy

Notes

_____

_____

_____

_____

_____

_____

My Period   *Month:_____*   *Year:_____*

Start	SUN	MON	TUE	WED	THU	FRI	SAT
End							
Day Length							
Next Period Expected							

Arrived:

☐ On Time ☐ Early ☐ Late

Feels:

☐ Normal ☐ See Doc

FLOW	1	2	3	4	5	6	7	8	9	10
Spotting	☐	☐	☐	☐	☐	☐	☐	☐	☐	☐
Light	☐	☐	☐	☐	☐	☐	☐	☐	☐	☐
Medium	☐	☐	☐	☐	☐	☐	☐	☐	☐	☐
Heavy	☐	☐	☐	☐	☐	☐	☐	☐	☐	☐
Ultra	☐	☐	☐	☐	☐	☐	☐	☐	☐	☐
PAIN 1	☐	☐	☐	☐	☐	☐	☐	☐	☐	☐
2	☐	☐	☐	☐	☐	☐	☐	☐	☐	☐
3	☐	☐	☐	☐	☐	☐	☐	☐	☐	☐
4	☐	☐	☐	☐	☐	☐	☐	☐	☐	☐
5	☐	☐	☐	☐	☐	☐	☐	☐	☐	☐

Period Symptoms

Discomfort: ☐ Cramps ☐ Mood Swings ☐ Headache ☐ Hunger ☐ Tender Breasts ☐ Back Pain ☐ Fatigue ☐ Acne ☐ Sleep Issues

Digestion: ☐ Nausea ☐ Ache ☐ Bloat ☐ Diarrhea ☐ Constipation

Cravings: ☐ Sweet ☐ Spice ☐ Salt ☐ Carb ☐ Cheese ☐ Alcohol

Emotions: ☐ Happy ☐ Energetic ☐ Motivated ☐ Calm ☐ Angry ☐ Irritated ☐ Sad ☐ Stressed ☐ Anxious ☐ Excited ☐ In Love

Body Check   Weight: _____

Exercise: ☐ Stretches ☐ Yoga ☐ Cardio ☐ Weights ☐ Impact

Diet: ☐ Healthy Eating ☐ Standard Diet ☐ Processed Food

Discharge Normal Colors: ☐ Clear ☐ White ☐ Pink ☐ Brown
NOT Normal: ☐ Yellow ☐ Green ☐ Gray ☐ White Lumps

Problems: ☐ Itchy ☐ Burning ☐ Soreness ☐ Weird Discharge ☐ Funky Smell ☐ Odd Changes ☐ Pain with Peeing ☐ Pain with Sex

Sex: ☐ Nope ☐ Solo ☐ Girls Only ☐ Protected ☐ Unprotected

Birth Control: ☐ Condom ☐ IUD ☐ Pill ☐ Patch ☐ Implant ☐ Shot ☐ Vaginal Ring ☐ Tubal Ligation ☐ Partner Vasectomy

Notes

_____

_____

_____

_____

_____

_____

My Period   *Month:_____*   *Year:_____*

Start	SUN	MON	TUE	WED	THU	FRI	SAT
End							
Day Length							
Next Period Expected							

Arrived:

☐ On Time ☐ Early ☐ Late

Feels:

☐ Normal ☐ See Doc

FLOW	1	2	3	4	5	6	7	8	9	10
Spotting	☐	☐	☐	☐	☐	☐	☐	☐	☐	☐
Light	☐	☐	☐	☐	☐	☐	☐	☐	☐	☐
Medium	☐	☐	☐	☐	☐	☐	☐	☐	☐	☐
Heavy	☐	☐	☐	☐	☐	☐	☐	☐	☐	☐
Ultra	☐	☐	☐	☐	☐	☐	☐	☐	☐	☐
PAIN 1	☐	☐	☐	☐	☐	☐	☐	☐	☐	☐
2	☐	☐	☐	☐	☐	☐	☐	☐	☐	☐
3	☐	☐	☐	☐	☐	☐	☐	☐	☐	☐
4	☐	☐	☐	☐	☐	☐	☐	☐	☐	☐
5	☐	☐	☐	☐	☐	☐	☐	☐	☐	☐

Period Symptoms

Discomfort: ☐ Cramps ☐ Mood Swings ☐ Headache ☐ Hunger
☐ Tender Breasts ☐ Back Pain ☐ Fatigue ☐ Acne ☐ Sleep Issues

Digestion: ☐ Nausea ☐ Ache ☐ Bloat ☐ Diarrhea ☐ Constipation

Cravings: ☐ Sweet ☐ Spice ☐ Salt ☐ Carb ☐ Cheese ☐ Alcohol

Emotions: ☐ Happy ☐ Energetic ☐ Motivated ☐ Calm ☐ Angry
☐ Irritated ☐ Sad ☐ Stressed ☐ Anxious ☐ Excited ☐ In Love

Body Check   Weight: _____

Exercise: ☐ Stretches ☐ Yoga ☐ Cardio ☐ Weights ☐ Impact

Diet: ☐ Healthy Eating ☐ Standard Diet ☐ Processed Food

Discharge Normal Colors: ☐ Clear ☐ White ☐ Pink ☐ Brown
  NOT Normal: ☐ Yellow ☐ Green ☐ Gray ☐ White Lumps

Problems: ☐ Itchy ☐ Burning ☐ Soreness ☐ Weird Discharge
☐ Funky Smell ☐ Odd Changes ☐ Pain with Peeing ☐ Pain with Sex

Sex: ☐ Nope ☐ Solo ☐ Girls Only ☐ Protected ☐ Unprotected

Birth Control: ☐ Condom ☐ IUD ☐ Pill ☐ Patch ☐ Implant
☐ Shot ☐ Vaginal Ring ☐ Tubal Ligation ☐ Partner Vasectomy

Notes

_____

_____

_____

_____

_____

_____

My Period   *Month:_____*   *Year:_____*

Start	SUN	MON	TUE	WED	THU	FRI	SAT

Start
[ ]

End
[ ]

Day Length
[ ]

Next Period Expected
[ ]

Arrived:

☐ On Time ☐ Early ☐ Late

Feels:

☐ Normal ☐ See Doc

FLOW	1	2	3	4	5	6	7	8	9	10
Spotting	☐	☐	☐	☐	☐	☐	☐	☐	☐	☐
Light	☐	☐	☐	☐	☐	☐	☐	☐	☐	☐
Medium	☐	☐	☐	☐	☐	☐	☐	☐	☐	☐
Heavy	☐	☐	☐	☐	☐	☐	☐	☐	☐	☐
Ultra	☐	☐	☐	☐	☐	☐	☐	☐	☐	☐
PAIN 1	☐	☐	☐	☐	☐	☐	☐	☐	☐	☐
2	☐	☐	☐	☐	☐	☐	☐	☐	☐	☐
3	☐	☐	☐	☐	☐	☐	☐	☐	☐	☐
4	☐	☐	☐	☐	☐	☐	☐	☐	☐	☐
5	☐	☐	☐	☐	☐	☐	☐	☐	☐	☐

Period Symptoms

Discomfort: ☐ Cramps ☐ Mood Swings ☐ Headache ☐ Hunger
☐ Tender Breasts ☐ Back Pain ☐ Fatigue ☐ Acne ☐ Sleep Issues

Digestion: ☐ Nausea ☐ Ache ☐ Bloat ☐ Diarrhea ☐ Constipation

Cravings: ☐ Sweet ☐ Spice ☐ Salt ☐ Carb ☐ Cheese ☐ Alcohol

Emotions: ☐ Happy ☐ Energetic ☐ Motivated ☐ Calm ☐ Angry
☐ Irritated ☐ Sad ☐ Stressed ☐ Anxious ☐ Excited ☐ In Love

Body Check   Weight: _____

Exercise: ☐ Stretches ☐ Yoga ☐ Cardio ☐ Weights ☐ Impact

Diet: ☐ Healthy Eating ☐ Standard Diet ☐ Processed Food

Discharge Normal Colors: ☐ Clear ☐ White ☐ Pink ☐ Brown
NOT Normal: ☐ Yellow ☐ Green ☐ Gray ☐ White Lumps

Problems: ☐ Itchy ☐ Burning ☐ Soreness ☐ Weird Discharge
☐ Funky Smell ☐ Odd Changes ☐ Pain with Peeing ☐ Pain with Sex

Sex: ☐ Nope ☐ Solo ☐ Girls Only ☐ Protected ☐ Unprotected

Birth Control: ☐ Condom ☐ IUD ☐ Pill ☐ Patch ☐ Implant
☐ Shot ☐ Vaginal Ring ☐ Tubal Ligation ☐ Partner Vasectomy

Notes

_____

_____

_____

_____

_____

_____

My Period *Month:*_____ *Year:*_____

Start	*SUN*	*MON*	*TUE*	*WED*	*THU*	*FRI*	*SAT*

End

Day Length

Next Period Expected

Arrived:

☐ On Time ☐ Early ☐ Late

Feels:

☐ Normal ☐ See Doc

FLOW	1	2	3	4	5	6	7	8	9	10
Spotting	☐	☐	☐	☐	☐	☐	☐	☐	☐	☐
Light	☐	☐	☐	☐	☐	☐	☐	☐	☐	☐
Medium	☐	☐	☐	☐	☐	☐	☐	☐	☐	☐
Heavy	☐	☐	☐	☐	☐	☐	☐	☐	☐	☐
Ultra	☐	☐	☐	☐	☐	☐	☐	☐	☐	☐
PAIN 1	☐	☐	☐	☐	☐	☐	☐	☐	☐	☐
2	☐	☐	☐	☐	☐	☐	☐	☐	☐	☐
3	☐	☐	☐	☐	☐	☐	☐	☐	☐	☐
4	☐	☐	☐	☐	☐	☐	☐	☐	☐	☐
5	☐	☐	☐	☐	☐	☐	☐	☐	☐	☐

Period Symptoms

Discomfort: ☐ Cramps ☐ Mood Swings ☐ Headache ☐ Hunger
☐ Tender Breasts ☐ Back Pain ☐ Fatigue ☐ Acne ☐ Sleep Issues

Digestion: ☐ Nausea ☐ Ache ☐ Bloat ☐ Diarrhea ☐ Constipation

Cravings: ☐ Sweet ☐ Spice ☐ Salt ☐ Carb ☐ Cheese ☐ Alcohol

Emotions: ☐ Happy ☐ Energetic ☐ Motivated ☐ Calm ☐ Angry
☐ Irritated ☐ Sad ☐ Stressed ☐ Anxious ☐ Excited ☐ In Love

Body Check   Weight: _____

Exercise: ☐ Stretches ☐ Yoga ☐ Cardio ☐ Weights ☐ Impact

Diet: ☐ Healthy Eating ☐ Standard Diet ☐ Processed Food

Discharge Normal Colors: ☐ Clear ☐ White ☐ Pink ☐ Brown
  NOT Normal: ☐ Yellow ☐ Green ☐ Gray ☐ White Lumps

Problems: ☐ Itchy ☐ Burning ☐ Soreness ☐ Weird Discharge
☐ Funky Smell ☐ Odd Changes ☐ Pain with Peeing ☐ Pain with Sex

Sex: ☐ Nope ☐ Solo ☐ Girls Only ☐ Protected ☐ Unprotected

Birth Control: ☐ Condom ☐ IUD ☐ Pill ☐ Patch ☐ Implant
☐ Shot ☐ Vaginal Ring ☐ Tubal Ligation ☐ Partner Vasectomy

Notes

_____

_____

_____

_____

_____

_____

My Period   *Month:*_____   *Year:*_____

Start	

	SUN	MON	TUE	WED	THU	FRI	SAT

End

Day Length

Next Period Expected

Arrived:

☐ On Time ☐ Early ☐ Late

Feels:

☐ Normal ☐ See Doc

FLOW	1	2	3	4	5	6	7	8	9	10
Spotting	☐	☐	☐	☐	☐	☐	☐	☐	☐	☐
Light	☐	☐	☐	☐	☐	☐	☐	☐	☐	☐
Medium	☐	☐	☐	☐	☐	☐	☐	☐	☐	☐
Heavy	☐	☐	☐	☐	☐	☐	☐	☐	☐	☐
Ultra	☐	☐	☐	☐	☐	☐	☐	☐	☐	☐
PAIN 1	☐	☐	☐	☐	☐	☐	☐	☐	☐	☐
2	☐	☐	☐	☐	☐	☐	☐	☐	☐	☐
3	☐	☐	☐	☐	☐	☐	☐	☐	☐	☐
4	☐	☐	☐	☐	☐	☐	☐	☐	☐	☐
5	☐	☐	☐	☐	☐	☐	☐	☐	☐	☐

Period Symptoms

Discomfort: ☐ Cramps ☐ Mood Swings ☐ Headache ☐ Hunger
☐ Tender Breasts ☐ Back Pain ☐ Fatigue ☐ Acne ☐ Sleep Issues

Digestion: ☐ Nausea ☐ Ache ☐ Bloat ☐ Diarrhea ☐ Constipation

Cravings: ☐ Sweet ☐ Spice ☐ Salt ☐ Carb ☐ Cheese ☐ Alcohol

Emotions: ☐ Happy ☐ Energetic ☐ Motivated ☐ Calm ☐ Angry
☐ Irritated ☐ Sad ☐ Stressed ☐ Anxious ☐ Excited ☐ In Love

Body Check   *Weight:* _____

Exercise: ☐ Stretches ☐ Yoga ☐ Cardio ☐ Weights ☐ Impact

Diet: ☐ Healthy Eating ☐ Standard Diet ☐ Processed Food

Discharge Normal Colors: ☐ Clear ☐ White ☐ Pink ☐ Brown
  NOT Normal: ☐ Yellow ☐ Green ☐ Gray ☐ White Lumps

Problems: ☐ Itchy ☐ Burning ☐ Soreness ☐ Weird Discharge
☐ Funky Smell ☐ Odd Changes ☐ Pain with Peeing ☐ Pain with Sex

Sex: ☐ Nope ☐ Solo ☐ Girls Only ☐ Protected ☐ Unprotected

Birth Control: ☐ Condom ☐ IUD ☐ Pill ☐ Patch ☐ Implant
☐ Shot ☐ Vaginal Ring ☐ Tubal Ligation ☐ Partner Vasectomy

Notes

_____

_____

_____

_____

_____

_____

My Period   *Month:_____*   *Year:_____*

Start	*SUN*	*MON*	*TUE*	*WED*	*THU*	*FRI*	*SAT*
End							
Day Length							
Next Period Expected							

Arrived:

☐ On Time ☐ Early ☐ Late

Feels:

☐ Normal ☐ See Doc

FLOW	1	2	3	4	5	6	7	8	9	10
Spotting	☐	☐	☐	☐	☐	☐	☐	☐	☐	☐
Light	☐	☐	☐	☐	☐	☐	☐	☐	☐	☐
Medium	☐	☐	☐	☐	☐	☐	☐	☐	☐	☐
Heavy	☐	☐	☐	☐	☐	☐	☐	☐	☐	☐
Ultra	☐	☐	☐	☐	☐	☐	☐	☐	☐	☐
PAIN 1	☐	☐	☐	☐	☐	☐	☐	☐	☐	☐
2	☐	☐	☐	☐	☐	☐	☐	☐	☐	☐
3	☐	☐	☐	☐	☐	☐	☐	☐	☐	☐
4	☐	☐	☐	☐	☐	☐	☐	☐	☐	☐
5	☐	☐	☐	☐	☐	☐	☐	☐	☐	☐

Period Symptoms

Discomfort: ☐ Cramps ☐ Mood Swings ☐ Headache ☐ Hunger
☐ Tender Breasts ☐ Back Pain ☐ Fatigue ☐ Acne ☐ Sleep Issues

Digestion: ☐ Nausea ☐ Ache ☐ Bloat ☐ Diarrhea ☐ Constipation

Cravings: ☐ Sweet ☐ Spice ☐ Salt ☐ Carb ☐ Cheese ☐ Alcohol

Emotions: ☐ Happy ☐ Energetic ☐ Motivated ☐ Calm ☐ Angry
☐ Irritated ☐ Sad ☐ Stressed ☐ Anxious ☐ Excited ☐ In Love

Body Check   *Weight:* _____

Exercise: ☐ Stretches ☐ Yoga ☐ Cardio ☐ Weights ☐ Impact

Diet: ☐ Healthy Eating ☐ Standard Diet ☐ Processed Food

Discharge Normal Colors: ☐ Clear ☐ White ☐ Pink ☐ Brown
    NOT Normal: ☐ Yellow ☐ Green ☐ Gray ☐ White Lumps

Problems: ☐ Itchy ☐ Burning ☐ Soreness ☐ Weird Discharge
☐ Funky Smell ☐ Odd Changes ☐ Pain with Peeing ☐ Pain with Sex

Sex: ☐ Nope ☐ Solo ☐ Girls Only ☐ Protected ☐ Unprotected

Birth Control: ☐ Condom ☐ IUD ☐ Pill ☐ Patch ☐ Implant
☐ Shot ☐ Vaginal Ring ☐ Tubal Ligation ☐ Partner Vasectomy

Notes

_____

_____

_____

_____

_____

_____

My Period   *Month:_____*   *Year:_____*

Start	SUN	MON	TUE	WED	THU	FRI	SAT

Start

End

Day Length

Next Period Expected

	SUN	MON	TUE	WED	THU	FRI	SAT

Arrived:

☐ On Time ☐ Early ☐ Late

Feels:

☐ Normal ☐ See Doc

FLOW	1	2	3	4	5	6	7	8	9	10
Spotting	☐	☐	☐	☐	☐	☐	☐	☐	☐	☐
Light	☐	☐	☐	☐	☐	☐	☐	☐	☐	☐
Medium	☐	☐	☐	☐	☐	☐	☐	☐	☐	☐
Heavy	☐	☐	☐	☐	☐	☐	☐	☐	☐	☐
Ultra	☐	☐	☐	☐	☐	☐	☐	☐	☐	☐
PAIN 1	☐	☐	☐	☐	☐	☐	☐	☐	☐	☐
2	☐	☐	☐	☐	☐	☐	☐	☐	☐	☐
3	☐	☐	☐	☐	☐	☐	☐	☐	☐	☐
4	☐	☐	☐	☐	☐	☐	☐	☐	☐	☐
5	☐	☐	☐	☐	☐	☐	☐	☐	☐	☐

Period Symptoms

Discomfort: ☐ Cramps ☐ Mood Swings ☐ Headache ☐ Hunger
☐ Tender Breasts ☐ Back Pain ☐ Fatigue ☐ Acne ☐ Sleep Issues

Digestion: ☐ Nausea ☐ Ache ☐ Bloat ☐ Diarrhea ☐ Constipation

Cravings: ☐ Sweet ☐ Spice ☐ Salt ☐ Carb ☐ Cheese ☐ Alcohol

Emotions: ☐ Happy ☐ Energetic ☐ Motivated ☐ Calm ☐ Angry
☐ Irritated ☐ Sad ☐ Stressed ☐ Anxious ☐ Excited ☐ In Love

Body Check   Weight: _____

Exercise: ☐ Stretches ☐ Yoga ☐ Cardio ☐ Weights ☐ Impact

Diet: ☐ Healthy Eating ☐ Standard Diet ☐ Processed Food

Discharge Normal Colors: ☐ Clear ☐ White ☐ Pink ☐ Brown
   NOT Normal: ☐ Yellow ☐ Green ☐ Gray ☐ White Lumps

Problems: ☐ Itchy ☐ Burning ☐ Soreness ☐ Weird Discharge
☐ Funky Smell ☐ Odd Changes ☐ Pain with Peeing ☐ Pain with Sex

Sex: ☐ Nope ☐ Solo ☐ Girls Only ☐ Protected ☐ Unprotected

Birth Control: ☐ Condom ☐ IUD ☐ Pill ☐ Patch ☐ Implant
☐ Shot ☐ Vaginal Ring ☐ Tubal Ligation ☐ Partner Vasectomy

Notes

_____

_____

_____

_____

_____

_____

My Period   *Month:_____*   *Year:_____*

Start	SUN	MON	TUE	WED	THU	FRI	SAT
End							
Day Length							
Next Period Expected							

Arrived:

☐ On Time ☐ Early ☐ Late

Feels:

☐ Normal ☐ See Doc

FLOW	1	2	3	4	5	6	7	8	9	10
Spotting	☐	☐	☐	☐	☐	☐	☐	☐	☐	☐
Light	☐	☐	☐	☐	☐	☐	☐	☐	☐	☐
Medium	☐	☐	☐	☐	☐	☐	☐	☐	☐	☐
Heavy	☐	☐	☐	☐	☐	☐	☐	☐	☐	☐
Ultra	☐	☐	☐	☐	☐	☐	☐	☐	☐	☐
PAIN 1	☐	☐	☐	☐	☐	☐	☐	☐	☐	☐
2	☐	☐	☐	☐	☐	☐	☐	☐	☐	☐
3	☐	☐	☐	☐	☐	☐	☐	☐	☐	☐
4	☐	☐	☐	☐	☐	☐	☐	☐	☐	☐
5	☐	☐	☐	☐	☐	☐	☐	☐	☐	☐

Period Symptoms

Discomfort: ☐ Cramps ☐ Mood Swings ☐ Headache ☐ Hunger
☐ Tender Breasts ☐ Back Pain ☐ Fatigue ☐ Acne ☐ Sleep Issues

Digestion: ☐ Nausea ☐ Ache ☐ Bloat ☐ Diarrhea ☐ Constipation

Cravings: ☐ Sweet ☐ Spice ☐ Salt ☐ Carb ☐ Cheese ☐ Alcohol

Emotions: ☐ Happy ☐ Energetic ☐ Motivated ☐ Calm ☐ Angry
☐ Irritated ☐ Sad ☐ Stressed ☐ Anxious ☐ Excited ☐ In Love

Body Check   Weight: _____

Exercise: ☐ Stretches ☐ Yoga ☐ Cardio ☐ Weights ☐ Impact

Diet: ☐ Healthy Eating ☐ Standard Diet ☐ Processed Food

Discharge Normal Colors: ☐ Clear ☐ White ☐ Pink ☐ Brown
NOT Normal: ☐ Yellow ☐ Green ☐ Gray ☐ White Lumps

Problems: ☐ Itchy ☐ Burning ☐ Soreness ☐ Weird Discharge
☐ Funky Smell ☐ Odd Changes ☐ Pain with Peeing ☐ Pain with Sex

Sex: ☐ Nope ☐ Solo ☐ Girls Only ☐ Protected ☐ Unprotected

Birth Control: ☐ Condom ☐ IUD ☐ Pill ☐ Patch ☐ Implant
☐ Shot ☐ Vaginal Ring ☐ Tubal Ligation ☐ Partner Vasectomy

Notes

_____

_____

_____

_____

_____

_____

My Period   *Month:_____*   *Year:_____*

Start	SUN	MON	TUE	WED	THU	FRI	SAT

End

Day Length

Next Period Expected

Arrived:

☐ On Time ☐ Early ☐ Late

Feels:

☐ Normal ☐ See Doc

FLOW	1	2	3	4	5	6	7	8	9	10
Spotting	☐	☐	☐	☐	☐	☐	☐	☐	☐	☐
Light	☐	☐	☐	☐	☐	☐	☐	☐	☐	☐
Medium	☐	☐	☐	☐	☐	☐	☐	☐	☐	☐
Heavy	☐	☐	☐	☐	☐	☐	☐	☐	☐	☐
Ultra	☐	☐	☐	☐	☐	☐	☐	☐	☐	☐
PAIN 1	☐	☐	☐	☐	☐	☐	☐	☐	☐	☐
2	☐	☐	☐	☐	☐	☐	☐	☐	☐	☐
3	☐	☐	☐	☐	☐	☐	☐	☐	☐	☐
4	☐	☐	☐	☐	☐	☐	☐	☐	☐	☐
5	☐	☐	☐	☐	☐	☐	☐	☐	☐	☐

Period Symptoms

Discomfort: ☐ Cramps ☐ Mood Swings ☐ Headache ☐ Hunger
☐ Tender Breasts ☐ Back Pain ☐ Fatigue ☐ Acne ☐ Sleep Issues

Digestion: ☐ Nausea ☐ Ache ☐ Bloat ☐ Diarrhea ☐ Constipation

Cravings: ☐ Sweet ☐ Spice ☐ Salt ☐ Carb ☐ Cheese ☐ Alcohol

Emotions: ☐ Happy ☐ Energetic ☐ Motivated ☐ Calm ☐ Angry
☐ Irritated ☐ Sad ☐ Stressed ☐ Anxious ☐ Excited ☐ In Love

Body Check   Weight: _____

Exercise: ☐ Stretches ☐ Yoga ☐ Cardio ☐ Weights ☐ Impact

Diet: ☐ Healthy Eating ☐ Standard Diet ☐ Processed Food

Discharge Normal Colors: ☐ Clear ☐ White ☐ Pink ☐ Brown
  NOT Normal: ☐ Yellow ☐ Green ☐ Gray ☐ White Lumps

Problems: ☐ Itchy ☐ Burning ☐ Soreness ☐ Weird Discharge
☐ Funky Smell ☐ Odd Changes ☐ Pain with Peeing ☐ Pain with Sex

Sex: ☐ Nope ☐ Solo ☐ Girls Only ☐ Protected ☐ Unprotected

Birth Control: ☐ Condom ☐ IUD ☐ Pill ☐ Patch ☐ Implant
☐ Shot ☐ Vaginal Ring ☐ Tubal Ligation ☐ Partner Vasectomy

Notes

_____

_____

_____

_____

_____

_____

My Period

Month:_____ Year:_____

Start	SUN	MON	TUE	WED	THU	FRI	SAT
End							
Day Length							
Next Period Expected							

Arrived:

☐ On Time ☐ Early ☐ Late

Feels:

☐ Normal ☐ See Doc

FLOW	1	2	3	4	5	6	7	8	9	10
Spotting	☐	☐	☐	☐	☐	☐	☐	☐	☐	☐
Light	☐	☐	☐	☐	☐	☐	☐	☐	☐	☐
Medium	☐	☐	☐	☐	☐	☐	☐	☐	☐	☐
Heavy	☐	☐	☐	☐	☐	☐	☐	☐	☐	☐
Ultra	☐	☐	☐	☐	☐	☐	☐	☐	☐	☐
PAIN 1	☐	☐	☐	☐	☐	☐	☐	☐	☐	☐
2	☐	☐	☐	☐	☐	☐	☐	☐	☐	☐
3	☐	☐	☐	☐	☐	☐	☐	☐	☐	☐
4	☐	☐	☐	☐	☐	☐	☐	☐	☐	☐
5	☐	☐	☐	☐	☐	☐	☐	☐	☐	☐

Period Symptoms

Discomfort: ☐ Cramps ☐ Mood Swings ☐ Headache ☐ Hunger
☐ Tender Breasts ☐ Back Pain ☐ Fatigue ☐ Acne ☐ Sleep Issues

Digestion: ☐ Nausea ☐ Ache ☐ Bloat ☐ Diarrhea ☐ Constipation

Cravings: ☐ Sweet ☐ Spice ☐ Salt ☐ Carb ☐ Cheese ☐ Alcohol

Emotions: ☐ Happy ☐ Energetic ☐ Motivated ☐ Calm ☐ Angry
☐ Irritated ☐ Sad ☐ Stressed ☐ Anxious ☐ Excited ☐ In Love

Body Check   *Weight:* _____

Exercise: ☐ Stretches ☐ Yoga ☐ Cardio ☐ Weights ☐ Impact

Diet: ☐ Healthy Eating ☐ Standard Diet ☐ Processed Food

Discharge Normal Colors: ☐ Clear ☐ White ☐ Pink ☐ Brown
   NOT Normal: ☐ Yellow ☐ Green ☐ Gray ☐ White Lumps

Problems: ☐ Itchy ☐ Burning ☐ Soreness ☐ Weird Discharge
☐ Funky Smell ☐ Odd Changes ☐ Pain with Peeing ☐ Pain with Sex

Sex: ☐ Nope ☐ Solo ☐ Girls Only ☐ Protected ☐ Unprotected

Birth Control: ☐ Condom ☐ IUD ☐ Pill ☐ Patch ☐ Implant
☐ Shot ☐ Vaginal Ring ☐ Tubal Ligation ☐ Partner Vasectomy

Notes

_____

_____

_____

_____

_____

_____

My Period *Month:_____* *Year:_____*

Start	*SUN*	*MON*	*TUE*	*WED*	*THU*	*FRI*	*SAT*
End							
Day Length							
Next Period Expected							

Arrived:

☐ On Time ☐ Early ☐ Late

Feels:

☐ Normal ☐ See Doc

FLOW	1	2	3	4	5	6	7	8	9	10
Spotting	☐	☐	☐	☐	☐	☐	☐	☐	☐	☐
Light	☐	☐	☐	☐	☐	☐	☐	☐	☐	☐
Medium	☐	☐	☐	☐	☐	☐	☐	☐	☐	☐
Heavy	☐	☐	☐	☐	☐	☐	☐	☐	☐	☐
Ultra	☐	☐	☐	☐	☐	☐	☐	☐	☐	☐
PAIN 1	☐	☐	☐	☐	☐	☐	☐	☐	☐	☐
2	☐	☐	☐	☐	☐	☐	☐	☐	☐	☐
3	☐	☐	☐	☐	☐	☐	☐	☐	☐	☐
4	☐	☐	☐	☐	☐	☐	☐	☐	☐	☐
5	☐	☐	☐	☐	☐	☐	☐	☐	☐	☐

Period Symptoms

Discomfort: ☐ Cramps ☐ Mood Swings ☐ Headache ☐ Hunger
☐ Tender Breasts ☐ Back Pain ☐ Fatigue ☐ Acne ☐ Sleep Issues

Digestion: ☐ Nausea ☐ Ache ☐ Bloat ☐ Diarrhea ☐ Constipation

Cravings: ☐ Sweet ☐ Spice ☐ Salt ☐ Carb ☐ Cheese ☐ Alcohol

Emotions: ☐ Happy ☐ Energetic ☐ Motivated ☐ Calm ☐ Angry
☐ Irritated ☐ Sad ☐ Stressed ☐ Anxious ☐ Excited ☐ In Love

Body Check   Weight: _____

Exercise: ☐ Stretches ☐ Yoga ☐ Cardio ☐ Weights ☐ Impact

Diet: ☐ Healthy Eating ☐ Standard Diet ☐ Processed Food

Discharge Normal Colors: ☐ Clear ☐ White ☐ Pink ☐ Brown
  NOT Normal: ☐ Yellow ☐ Green ☐ Gray ☐ White Lumps

Problems: ☐ Itchy ☐ Burning ☐ Soreness ☐ Weird Discharge
☐ Funky Smell ☐ Odd Changes ☐ Pain with Peeing ☐ Pain with Sex

Sex: ☐ Nope ☐ Solo ☐ Girls Only ☐ Protected ☐ Unprotected

Birth Control: ☐ Condom ☐ IUD ☐ Pill ☐ Patch ☐ Implant
☐ Shot ☐ Vaginal Ring ☐ Tubal Ligation ☐ Partner Vasectomy

Notes

_____

_____

_____

_____

_____

_____

My Period

Month:_____   *Year:_____*

Start	SUN	MON	TUE	WED	THU	FRI	SAT
End							
Day Length							
Next Period Expected							

Arrived:

☐ On Time ☐ Early ☐ Late

Feels:

☐ Normal ☐ See Doc

FLOW	1	2	3	4	5	6	7	8	9	10
Spotting	☐	☐	☐	☐	☐	☐	☐	☐	☐	☐
Light	☐	☐	☐	☐	☐	☐	☐	☐	☐	☐
Medium	☐	☐	☐	☐	☐	☐	☐	☐	☐	☐
Heavy	☐	☐	☐	☐	☐	☐	☐	☐	☐	☐
Ultra	☐	☐	☐	☐	☐	☐	☐	☐	☐	☐
PAIN 1	☐	☐	☐	☐	☐	☐	☐	☐	☐	☐
2	☐	☐	☐	☐	☐	☐	☐	☐	☐	☐
3	☐	☐	☐	☐	☐	☐	☐	☐	☐	☐
4	☐	☐	☐	☐	☐	☐	☐	☐	☐	☐
5	☐	☐	☐	☐	☐	☐	☐	☐	☐	☐

Period Symptoms

Discomfort: ☐ Cramps ☐ Mood Swings ☐ Headache ☐ Hunger ☐ Tender Breasts ☐ Back Pain ☐ Fatigue ☐ Acne ☐ Sleep Issues

Digestion: ☐ Nausea ☐ Ache ☐ Bloat ☐ Diarrhea ☐ Constipation

Cravings: ☐ Sweet ☐ Spice ☐ Salt ☐ Carb ☐ Cheese ☐ Alcohol

Emotions: ☐ Happy ☐ Energetic ☐ Motivated ☐ Calm ☐ Angry ☐ Irritated ☐ Sad ☐ Stressed ☐ Anxious ☐ Excited ☐ In Love

Body Check   *Weight:* _____

Exercise: ☐ Stretches ☐ Yoga ☐ Cardio ☐ Weights ☐ Impact

Diet: ☐ Healthy Eating ☐ Standard Diet ☐ Processed Food

Discharge Normal Colors: ☐ Clear ☐ White ☐ Pink ☐ Brown **NOT Normal:** ☐ Yellow ☐ Green ☐ Gray ☐ White Lumps

Problems: ☐ Itchy ☐ Burning ☐ Soreness ☐ Weird Discharge ☐ Funky Smell ☐ Odd Changes ☐ Pain with Peeing ☐ Pain with Sex

Sex: ☐ Nope ☐ Solo ☐ Girls Only ☐ Protected ☐ Unprotected

Birth Control: ☐ Condom ☐ IUD ☐ Pill ☐ Patch ☐ Implant ☐ Shot ☐ Vaginal Ring ☐ Tubal Ligation ☐ Partner Vasectomy

Notes

_____

_____

_____

_____

_____

_____

My Period   *Month:*_____   *Year:*_____

Start	SUN	MON	TUE	WED	THU	FRI	SAT
End							
Day Length							
Next Period Expected							

Arrived:

☐ On Time ☐ Early ☐ Late

Feels:

☐ Normal ☐ See Doc

FLOW	1	2	3	4	5	6	7	8	9	10
Spotting	☐	☐	☐	☐	☐	☐	☐	☐	☐	☐
Light	☐	☐	☐	☐	☐	☐	☐	☐	☐	☐
Medium	☐	☐	☐	☐	☐	☐	☐	☐	☐	☐
Heavy	☐	☐	☐	☐	☐	☐	☐	☐	☐	☐
Ultra	☐	☐	☐	☐	☐	☐	☐	☐	☐	☐
PAIN 1	☐	☐	☐	☐	☐	☐	☐	☐	☐	☐
2	☐	☐	☐	☐	☐	☐	☐	☐	☐	☐
3	☐	☐	☐	☐	☐	☐	☐	☐	☐	☐
4	☐	☐	☐	☐	☐	☐	☐	☐	☐	☐
5	☐	☐	☐	☐	☐	☐	☐	☐	☐	☐

Period Symptoms

Discomfort: ☐ Cramps ☐ Mood Swings ☐ Headache ☐ Hunger
☐ Tender Breasts ☐ Back Pain ☐ Fatigue ☐ Acne ☐ Sleep Issues

Digestion: ☐ Nausea ☐ Ache ☐ Bloat ☐ Diarrhea ☐ Constipation

Cravings: ☐ Sweet ☐ Spice ☐ Salt ☐ Carb ☐ Cheese ☐ Alcohol

Emotions: ☐ Happy ☐ Energetic ☐ Motivated ☐ Calm ☐ Angry
☐ Irritated ☐ Sad ☐ Stressed ☐ Anxious ☐ Excited ☐ In Love

Body Check   *Weight:* _____

Exercise: ☐ Stretches ☐ Yoga ☐ Cardio ☐ Weights ☐ Impact

Diet: ☐ Healthy Eating ☐ Standard Diet ☐ Processed Food

Discharge Normal Colors: ☐ Clear ☐ White ☐ Pink ☐ Brown
   NOT Normal: ☐ Yellow ☐ Green ☐ Gray ☐ White Lumps

Problems: ☐ Itchy ☐ Burning ☐ Soreness ☐ Weird Discharge
☐ Funky Smell ☐ Odd Changes ☐ Pain with Peeing ☐ Pain with Sex

Sex: ☐ Nope ☐ Solo ☐ Girls Only ☐ Protected ☐ Unprotected

Birth Control: ☐ Condom ☐ IUD ☐ Pill ☐ Patch ☐ Implant
☐ Shot ☐ Vaginal Ring ☐ Tubal Ligation ☐ Partner Vasectomy

Notes

_____

_____

_____

_____

_____

_____

My Period   *Month:_____   Year:_____*

Start	SUN	MON	TUE	WED	THU	FRI	SAT
End							
Day Length							
Next Period Expected							

Arrived:

☐ On Time ☐ Early ☐ Late

Feels:

☐ Normal ☐ See Doc

FLOW	1	2	3	4	5	6	7	8	9	10
Spotting	☐	☐	☐	☐	☐	☐	☐	☐	☐	☐
Light	☐	☐	☐	☐	☐	☐	☐	☐	☐	☐
Medium	☐	☐	☐	☐	☐	☐	☐	☐	☐	☐
Heavy	☐	☐	☐	☐	☐	☐	☐	☐	☐	☐
Ultra	☐	☐	☐	☐	☐	☐	☐	☐	☐	☐
PAIN 1	☐	☐	☐	☐	☐	☐	☐	☐	☐	☐
2	☐	☐	☐	☐	☐	☐	☐	☐	☐	☐
3	☐	☐	☐	☐	☐	☐	☐	☐	☐	☐
4	☐	☐	☐	☐	☐	☐	☐	☐	☐	☐
5	☐	☐	☐	☐	☐	☐	☐	☐	☐	☐

Period Symptoms

Discomfort: ☐ Cramps ☐ Mood Swings ☐ Headache ☐ Hunger
☐ Tender Breasts ☐ Back Pain ☐ Fatigue ☐ Acne ☐ Sleep Issues

Digestion: ☐ Nausea ☐ Ache ☐ Bloat ☐ Diarrhea ☐ Constipation

Cravings: ☐ Sweet ☐ Spice ☐ Salt ☐ Carb ☐ Cheese ☐ Alcohol

Emotions: ☐ Happy ☐ Energetic ☐ Motivated ☐ Calm ☐ Angry
☐ Irritated ☐ Sad ☐ Stressed ☐ Anxious ☐ Excited ☐ In Love

Body Check   Weight: _____

Exercise: ☐ Stretches ☐ Yoga ☐ Cardio ☐ Weights ☐ Impact

Diet: ☐ Healthy Eating ☐ Standard Diet ☐ Processed Food

Discharge Normal Colors: ☐ Clear ☐ White ☐ Pink ☐ Brown
NOT Normal: ☐ Yellow ☐ Green ☐ Gray ☐ White Lumps

Problems: ☐ Itchy ☐ Burning ☐ Soreness ☐ Weird Discharge
☐ Funky Smell ☐ Odd Changes ☐ Pain with Peeing ☐ Pain with Sex

Sex: ☐ Nope ☐ Solo ☐ Girls Only ☐ Protected ☐ Unprotected

Birth Control: ☐ Condom ☐ IUD ☐ Pill ☐ Patch ☐ Implant
☐ Shot ☐ Vaginal Ring ☐ Tubal Ligation ☐ Partner Vasectomy

Notes

_____

_____

_____

_____

_____

_____

My Period   *Month:_____*   *Year:_____*

Start	SUN	MON	TUE	WED	THU	FRI	SAT
End							
Day Length							
Next Period Expected							

Arrived:

☐ On Time ☐ Early ☐ Late

Feels:

☐ Normal ☐ See Doc

FLOW	1	2	3	4	5	6	7	8	9	10
Spotting	☐	☐	☐	☐	☐	☐	☐	☐	☐	☐
Light	☐	☐	☐	☐	☐	☐	☐	☐	☐	☐
Medium	☐	☐	☐	☐	☐	☐	☐	☐	☐	☐
Heavy	☐	☐	☐	☐	☐	☐	☐	☐	☐	☐
Ultra	☐	☐	☐	☐	☐	☐	☐	☐	☐	☐
PAIN 1	☐	☐	☐	☐	☐	☐	☐	☐	☐	☐
2	☐	☐	☐	☐	☐	☐	☐	☐	☐	☐
3	☐	☐	☐	☐	☐	☐	☐	☐	☐	☐
4	☐	☐	☐	☐	☐	☐	☐	☐	☐	☐
5	☐	☐	☐	☐	☐	☐	☐	☐	☐	☐

Period Symptoms

Discomfort: ☐ Cramps ☐ Mood Swings ☐ Headache ☐ Hunger
☐ Tender Breasts ☐ Back Pain ☐ Fatigue ☐ Acne ☐ Sleep Issues

Digestion: ☐ Nausea ☐ Ache ☐ Bloat ☐ Diarrhea ☐ Constipation

Cravings: ☐ Sweet ☐ Spice ☐ Salt ☐ Carb ☐ Cheese ☐ Alcohol

Emotions: ☐ Happy ☐ Energetic ☐ Motivated ☐ Calm ☐ Angry
☐ Irritated ☐ Sad ☐ Stressed ☐ Anxious ☐ Excited ☐ In Love

Body Check   *Weight:* _____

Exercise: ☐ Stretches ☐ Yoga ☐ Cardio ☐ Weights ☐ Impact

Diet: ☐ Healthy Eating ☐ Standard Diet ☐ Processed Food

Discharge Normal Colors: ☐ Clear ☐ White ☐ Pink ☐ Brown
  NOT Normal: ☐ Yellow ☐ Green ☐ Gray ☐ White Lumps

Problems: ☐ Itchy ☐ Burning ☐ Soreness ☐ Weird Discharge
☐ Funky Smell ☐ Odd Changes ☐ Pain with Peeing ☐ Pain with Sex

Sex: ☐ Nope ☐ Solo ☐ Girls Only ☐ Protected ☐ Unprotected

Birth Control: ☐ Condom ☐ IUD ☐ Pill ☐ Patch ☐ Implant
☐ Shot ☐ Vaginal Ring ☐ Tubal Ligation ☐ Partner Vasectomy

Notes

_____

_____

_____

_____

_____

_____

My Period   *Month:*_____   *Year:*_____

Start	*SUN*	*MON*	*TUE*	*WED*	*THU*	*FRI*	*SAT*

End

Day Length

Next Period Expected

Arrived:

☐ On Time ☐ Early ☐ Late

Feels:

☐ Normal ☐ See Doc

FLOW	1	2	3	4	5	6	7	8	9	10
Spotting	☐	☐	☐	☐	☐	☐	☐	☐	☐	☐
Light	☐	☐	☐	☐	☐	☐	☐	☐	☐	☐
Medium	☐	☐	☐	☐	☐	☐	☐	☐	☐	☐
Heavy	☐	☐	☐	☐	☐	☐	☐	☐	☐	☐
Ultra	☐	☐	☐	☐	☐	☐	☐	☐	☐	☐
PAIN 1	☐	☐	☐	☐	☐	☐	☐	☐	☐	☐
2	☐	☐	☐	☐	☐	☐	☐	☐	☐	☐
3	☐	☐	☐	☐	☐	☐	☐	☐	☐	☐
4	☐	☐	☐	☐	☐	☐	☐	☐	☐	☐
5	☐	☐	☐	☐	☐	☐	☐	☐	☐	☐

Period Symptoms

Discomfort: ☐ Cramps ☐ Mood Swings ☐ Headache ☐ Hunger
☐ Tender Breasts ☐ Back Pain ☐ Fatigue ☐ Acne ☐ Sleep Issues

Digestion: ☐ Nausea ☐ Ache ☐ Bloat ☐ Diarrhea ☐ Constipation

Cravings: ☐ Sweet ☐ Spice ☐ Salt ☐ Carb ☐ Cheese ☐ Alcohol

Emotions: ☐ Happy ☐ Energetic ☐ Motivated ☐ Calm ☐ Angry
☐ Irritated ☐ Sad ☐ Stressed ☐ Anxious ☐ Excited ☐ In Love

Body Check   *Weight:* _____

Exercise: ☐ Stretches ☐ Yoga ☐ Cardio ☐ Weights ☐ Impact

Diet: ☐ Healthy Eating ☐ Standard Diet ☐ Processed Food

Discharge Normal Colors: ☐ Clear ☐ White ☐ Pink ☐ Brown
NOT Normal: ☐ Yellow ☐ Green ☐ Gray ☐ White Lumps

Problems: ☐ Itchy ☐ Burning ☐ Soreness ☐ Weird Discharge
☐ Funky Smell ☐ Odd Changes ☐ Pain with Peeing ☐ Pain with Sex

Sex: ☐ Nope ☐ Solo ☐ Girls Only ☐ Protected ☐ Unprotected

Birth Control: ☐ Condom ☐ IUD ☐ Pill ☐ Patch ☐ Implant
☐ Shot ☐ Vaginal Ring ☐ Tubal Ligation ☐ Partner Vasectomy

Notes

_____

_____

_____

_____

_____

_____

My Period

Month:_____ **Year:**_____

	SUN	MON	TUE	WED	THU	FRI	SAT

Start

End

Day Length

Next Period Expected

Arrived:

☐ On Time ☐ Early ☐ Late

Feels:

☐ Normal ☐ See Doc

FLOW	1	2	3	4	5	6	7	8	9	10
Spotting	☐	☐	☐	☐	☐	☐	☐	☐	☐	☐
Light	☐	☐	☐	☐	☐	☐	☐	☐	☐	☐
Medium	☐	☐	☐	☐	☐	☐	☐	☐	☐	☐
Heavy	☐	☐	☐	☐	☐	☐	☐	☐	☐	☐
Ultra	☐	☐	☐	☐	☐	☐	☐	☐	☐	☐
PAIN 1	☐	☐	☐	☐	☐	☐	☐	☐	☐	☐
2	☐	☐	☐	☐	☐	☐	☐	☐	☐	☐
3	☐	☐	☐	☐	☐	☐	☐	☐	☐	☐
4	☐	☐	☐	☐	☐	☐	☐	☐	☐	☐
5	☐	☐	☐	☐	☐	☐	☐	☐	☐	☐

Period Symptoms

Discomfort: ☐ Cramps ☐ Mood Swings ☐ Headache ☐ Hunger
☐ Tender Breasts ☐ Back Pain ☐ Fatigue ☐ Acne ☐ Sleep Issues

Digestion: ☐ Nausea ☐ Ache ☐ Bloat ☐ Diarrhea ☐ Constipation

Cravings: ☐ Sweet ☐ Spice ☐ Salt ☐ Carb ☐ Cheese ☐ Alcohol

Emotions: ☐ Happy ☐ Energetic ☐ Motivated ☐ Calm ☐ Angry
☐ Irritated ☐ Sad ☐ Stressed ☐ Anxious ☐ Excited ☐ In Love

Body Check   *Weight:* _____

Exercise: ☐ Stretches ☐ Yoga ☐ Cardio ☐ Weights ☐ Impact

Diet: ☐ Healthy Eating ☐ Standard Diet ☐ Processed Food

Discharge Normal Colors: ☐ Clear ☐ White ☐ Pink ☐ Brown
  NOT Normal: ☐ Yellow ☐ Green ☐ Gray ☐ White Lumps

Problems: ☐ Itchy ☐ Burning ☐ Soreness ☐ Weird Discharge
☐ Funky Smell ☐ Odd Changes ☐ Pain with Peeing ☐ Pain with Sex

Sex: ☐ Nope ☐ Solo ☐ Girls Only ☐ Protected ☐ Unprotected

Birth Control: ☐ Condom ☐ IUD ☐ Pill ☐ Patch ☐ Implant
☐ Shot ☐ Vaginal Ring ☐ Tubal Ligation ☐ Partner Vasectomy

Notes

_____

_____

_____

_____

_____

_____

My Period

*Month:*_____ *Year:*_____

Start	SUN	MON	TUE	WED	THU	FRI	SAT
End							
Day Length							
Next Period Expected							

Arrived:

☐ On Time ☐ Early ☐ Late

Feels:

☐ Normal ☐ See Doc

FLOW	1	2	3	4	5	6	7	8	9	10
Spotting	☐	☐	☐	☐	☐	☐	☐	☐	☐	☐
Light	☐	☐	☐	☐	☐	☐	☐	☐	☐	☐
Medium	☐	☐	☐	☐	☐	☐	☐	☐	☐	☐
Heavy	☐	☐	☐	☐	☐	☐	☐	☐	☐	☐
Ultra	☐	☐	☐	☐	☐	☐	☐	☐	☐	☐
PAIN 1	☐	☐	☐	☐	☐	☐	☐	☐	☐	☐
2	☐	☐	☐	☐	☐	☐	☐	☐	☐	☐
3	☐	☐	☐	☐	☐	☐	☐	☐	☐	☐
4	☐	☐	☐	☐	☐	☐	☐	☐	☐	☐
5	☐	☐	☐	☐	☐	☐	☐	☐	☐	☐

Period Symptoms

Discomfort: ☐ Cramps ☐ Mood Swings ☐ Headache ☐ Hunger ☐ Tender Breasts ☐ Back Pain ☐ Fatigue ☐ Acne ☐ Sleep Issues

Digestion: ☐ Nausea ☐ Ache ☐ Bloat ☐ Diarrhea ☐ Constipation

Cravings: ☐ Sweet ☐ Spice ☐ Salt ☐ Carb ☐ Cheese ☐ Alcohol

Emotions: ☐ Happy ☐ Energetic ☐ Motivated ☐ Calm ☐ Angry ☐ Irritated ☐ Sad ☐ Stressed ☐ Anxious ☐ Excited ☐ In Love

Body Check   Weight: _____

Exercise: ☐ Stretches ☐ Yoga ☐ Cardio ☐ Weights ☐ Impact

Diet: ☐ Healthy Eating ☐ Standard Diet ☐ Processed Food

Discharge Normal Colors: ☐ Clear ☐ White ☐ Pink ☐ Brown **NOT Normal:** ☐ Yellow ☐ Green ☐ Gray ☐ White Lumps

Problems: ☐ Itchy ☐ Burning ☐ Soreness ☐ Weird Discharge ☐ Funky Smell ☐ Odd Changes ☐ Pain with Peeing ☐ Pain with Sex

Sex: ☐ Nope ☐ Solo ☐ Girls Only ☐ Protected ☐ Unprotected

Birth Control: ☐ Condom ☐ IUD ☐ Pill ☐ Patch ☐ Implant ☐ Shot ☐ Vaginal Ring ☐ Tubal Ligation ☐ Partner Vasectomy

Notes

_____

_____

_____

_____

_____

_____

My Period

Month:_____ Year:_____

Start

| | | | | | | |
SUN	MON	TUE	WED	THU	FRI	SAT

End

Day Length

Next Period Expected

Arrived:

☐ On Time ☐ Early ☐ Late

Feels:

☐ Normal ☐ See Doc

FLOW	1	2	3	4	5	6	7	8	9	10
Spotting	☐	☐	☐	☐	☐	☐	☐	☐	☐	☐
Light	☐	☐	☐	☐	☐	☐	☐	☐	☐	☐
Medium	☐	☐	☐	☐	☐	☐	☐	☐	☐	☐
Heavy	☐	☐	☐	☐	☐	☐	☐	☐	☐	☐
Ultra	☐	☐	☐	☐	☐	☐	☐	☐	☐	☐
PAIN 1	☐	☐	☐	☐	☐	☐	☐	☐	☐	☐
2	☐	☐	☐	☐	☐	☐	☐	☐	☐	☐
3	☐	☐	☐	☐	☐	☐	☐	☐	☐	☐
4	☐	☐	☐	☐	☐	☐	☐	☐	☐	☐
5	☐	☐	☐	☐	☐	☐	☐	☐	☐	☐

Period Symptoms

Discomfort: ☐ Cramps ☐ Mood Swings ☐ Headache ☐ Hunger
☐ Tender Breasts ☐ Back Pain ☐ Fatigue ☐ Acne ☐ Sleep Issues

Digestion: ☐ Nausea ☐ Ache ☐ Bloat ☐ Diarrhea ☐ Constipation

Cravings: ☐ Sweet ☐ Spice ☐ Salt ☐ Carb ☐ Cheese ☐ Alcohol

Emotions: ☐ Happy ☐ Energetic ☐ Motivated ☐ Calm ☐ Angry
☐ Irritated ☐ Sad ☐ Stressed ☐ Anxious ☐ Excited ☐ In Love

Body Check   *Weight:* _____

Exercise: ☐ Stretches ☐ Yoga ☐ Cardio ☐ Weights ☐ Impact

Diet: ☐ Healthy Eating ☐ Standard Diet ☐ Processed Food

Discharge Normal Colors: ☐ Clear ☐ White ☐ Pink ☐ Brown
 NOT Normal: ☐ Yellow ☐ Green ☐ Gray ☐ White Lumps

Problems: ☐ Itchy ☐ Burning ☐ Soreness ☐ Weird Discharge
☐ Funky Smell ☐ Odd Changes ☐ Pain with Peeing ☐ Pain with Sex

Sex: ☐ Nope ☐ Solo ☐ Girls Only ☐ Protected ☐ Unprotected

Birth Control: ☐ Condom ☐ IUD ☐ Pill ☐ Patch ☐ Implant
☐ Shot ☐ Vaginal Ring ☐ Tubal Ligation ☐ Partner Vasectomy

Notes

_____

_____

_____

_____

_____

_____

My Period

*Month:*_____ *Year:*_____

Start	SUN	MON	TUE	WED	THU	FRI	SAT

End

Day Length

Next Period Expected

Arrived:

☐ On Time ☐ Early ☐ Late

Feels:

☐ Normal ☐ See Doc

FLOW	1	2	3	4	5	6	7	8	9	10
Spotting	☐	☐	☐	☐	☐	☐	☐	☐	☐	☐
Light	☐	☐	☐	☐	☐	☐	☐	☐	☐	☐
Medium	☐	☐	☐	☐	☐	☐	☐	☐	☐	☐
Heavy	☐	☐	☐	☐	☐	☐	☐	☐	☐	☐
Ultra	☐	☐	☐	☐	☐	☐	☐	☐	☐	☐
PAIN 1	☐	☐	☐	☐	☐	☐	☐	☐	☐	☐
2	☐	☐	☐	☐	☐	☐	☐	☐	☐	☐
3	☐	☐	☐	☐	☐	☐	☐	☐	☐	☐
4	☐	☐	☐	☐	☐	☐	☐	☐	☐	☐
5	☐	☐	☐	☐	☐	☐	☐	☐	☐	☐

Period Symptoms

Discomfort: ☐ Cramps ☐ Mood Swings ☐ Headache ☐ Hunger
☐ Tender Breasts ☐ Back Pain ☐ Fatigue ☐ Acne ☐ Sleep Issues

Digestion: ☐ Nausea ☐ Ache ☐ Bloat ☐ Diarrhea ☐ Constipation

Cravings: ☐ Sweet ☐ Spice ☐ Salt ☐ Carb ☐ Cheese ☐ Alcohol

Emotions: ☐ Happy ☐ Energetic ☐ Motivated ☐ Calm ☐ Angry
☐ Irritated ☐ Sad ☐ Stressed ☐ Anxious ☐ Excited ☐ In Love

Body Check   *Weight:* _____

Exercise: ☐ Stretches ☐ Yoga ☐ Cardio ☐ Weights ☐ Impact

Diet: ☐ Healthy Eating ☐ Standard Diet ☐ Processed Food

Discharge Normal Colors: ☐ Clear ☐ White ☐ Pink ☐ Brown
NOT Normal: ☐ Yellow ☐ Green ☐ Gray ☐ White Lumps

Problems: ☐ Itchy ☐ Burning ☐ Soreness ☐ Weird Discharge
☐ Funky Smell ☐ Odd Changes ☐ Pain with Peeing ☐ Pain with Sex

Sex: ☐ Nope ☐ Solo ☐ Girls Only ☐ Protected ☐ Unprotected

Birth Control: ☐ Condom ☐ IUD ☐ Pill ☐ Patch ☐ Implant
☐ Shot ☐ Vaginal Ring ☐ Tubal Ligation ☐ Partner Vasectomy

Notes

_____

_____

_____

_____

_____

_____

My Period   *Month:_____*   *Year:_____*

	SUN	MON	TUE	WED	THU	FRI	SAT
Start							
End							
Day Length							
Next Period Expected							

Start

End

Day Length

Next Period Expected

Arrived:

☐ On Time ☐ Early ☐ Late

Feels:

☐ Normal ☐ See Doc

FLOW	1	2	3	4	5	6	7	8	9	10
Spotting	☐	☐	☐	☐	☐	☐	☐	☐	☐	☐
Light	☐	☐	☐	☐	☐	☐	☐	☐	☐	☐
Medium	☐	☐	☐	☐	☐	☐	☐	☐	☐	☐
Heavy	☐	☐	☐	☐	☐	☐	☐	☐	☐	☐
Ultra	☐	☐	☐	☐	☐	☐	☐	☐	☐	☐
PAIN 1	☐	☐	☐	☐	☐	☐	☐	☐	☐	☐
2	☐	☐	☐	☐	☐	☐	☐	☐	☐	☐
3	☐	☐	☐	☐	☐	☐	☐	☐	☐	☐
4	☐	☐	☐	☐	☐	☐	☐	☐	☐	☐
5	☐	☐	☐	☐	☐	☐	☐	☐	☐	☐

Period Symptoms

Discomfort: ☐ Cramps ☐ Mood Swings ☐ Headache ☐ Hunger
☐ Tender Breasts ☐ Back Pain ☐ Fatigue ☐ Acne ☐ Sleep Issues

Digestion: ☐ Nausea ☐ Ache ☐ Bloat ☐ Diarrhea ☐ Constipation

Cravings: ☐ Sweet ☐ Spice ☐ Salt ☐ Carb ☐ Cheese ☐ Alcohol

Emotions: ☐ Happy ☐ Energetic ☐ Motivated ☐ Calm ☐ Angry
☐ Irritated ☐ Sad ☐ Stressed ☐ Anxious ☐ Excited ☐ In Love

Body Check   *Weight:* _____

Exercise: ☐ Stretches ☐ Yoga ☐ Cardio ☐ Weights ☐ Impact

Diet: ☐ Healthy Eating ☐ Standard Diet ☐ Processed Food

Discharge Normal Colors: ☐ Clear ☐ White ☐ Pink ☐ Brown
   NOT Normal: ☐ Yellow ☐ Green ☐ Gray ☐ White Lumps

Problems: ☐ Itchy ☐ Burning ☐ Soreness ☐ Weird Discharge
☐ Funky Smell ☐ Odd Changes ☐ Pain with Peeing ☐ Pain with Sex

Sex: ☐ Nope ☐ Solo ☐ Girls Only ☐ Protected ☐ Unprotected

Birth Control: ☐ Condom ☐ IUD ☐ Pill ☐ Patch ☐ Implant
☐ Shot ☐ Vaginal Ring ☐ Tubal Ligation ☐ Partner Vasectomy

Notes

_____

_____

_____

_____

_____

_____

My Period   *Month:_____   Year:_____*

Start	SUN	MON	TUE	WED	THU	FRI	SAT

End

Day Length

Next Period Expected

Arrived:

☐ On Time ☐ Early ☐ Late

Feels:

☐ Normal ☐ See Doc

FLOW	1	2	3	4	5	6	7	8	9	10
Spotting	☐	☐	☐	☐	☐	☐	☐	☐	☐	☐
Light	☐	☐	☐	☐	☐	☐	☐	☐	☐	☐
Medium	☐	☐	☐	☐	☐	☐	☐	☐	☐	☐
Heavy	☐	☐	☐	☐	☐	☐	☐	☐	☐	☐
Ultra	☐	☐	☐	☐	☐	☐	☐	☐	☐	☐
PAIN 1	☐	☐	☐	☐	☐	☐	☐	☐	☐	☐
2	☐	☐	☐	☐	☐	☐	☐	☐	☐	☐
3	☐	☐	☐	☐	☐	☐	☐	☐	☐	☐
4	☐	☐	☐	☐	☐	☐	☐	☐	☐	☐
5	☐	☐	☐	☐	☐	☐	☐	☐	☐	☐

Period Symptoms

Discomfort: ☐ Cramps ☐ Mood Swings ☐ Headache ☐ Hunger
☐ Tender Breasts ☐ Back Pain ☐ Fatigue ☐ Acne ☐ Sleep Issues

Digestion: ☐ Nausea ☐ Ache ☐ Bloat ☐ Diarrhea ☐ Constipation

Cravings: ☐ Sweet ☐ Spice ☐ Salt ☐ Carb ☐ Cheese ☐ Alcohol

Emotions: ☐ Happy ☐ Energetic ☐ Motivated ☐ Calm ☐ Angry
☐ Irritated ☐ Sad ☐ Stressed ☐ Anxious ☐ Excited ☐ In Love

Body Check   Weight: _____

Exercise: ☐ Stretches ☐ Yoga ☐ Cardio ☐ Weights ☐ Impact

Diet: ☐ Healthy Eating ☐ Standard Diet ☐ Processed Food

Discharge Normal Colors: ☐ Clear ☐ White ☐ Pink ☐ Brown
NOT Normal: ☐ Yellow ☐ Green ☐ Gray ☐ White Lumps

Problems: ☐ Itchy ☐ Burning ☐ Soreness ☐ Weird Discharge
☐ Funky Smell ☐ Odd Changes ☐ Pain with Peeing ☐ Pain with Sex

Sex: ☐ Nope ☐ Solo ☐ Girls Only ☐ Protected ☐ Unprotected

Birth Control: ☐ Condom ☐ IUD ☐ Pill ☐ Patch ☐ Implant
☐ Shot ☐ Vaginal Ring ☐ Tubal Ligation ☐ Partner Vasectomy

Notes

_____

_____

_____

_____

_____

_____

My Period

Month:_____ **Year:**_____

		SUN	MON	TUE	WED	THU	FRI	SAT

Start

End

Day Length

Next Period Expected

Arrived:

☐ On Time ☐ Early ☐ Late

Feels:

☐ Normal ☐ See Doc

FLOW	1	2	3	4	5	6	7	8	9	10
Spotting	☐	☐	☐	☐	☐	☐	☐	☐	☐	☐
Light	☐	☐	☐	☐	☐	☐	☐	☐	☐	☐
Medium	☐	☐	☐	☐	☐	☐	☐	☐	☐	☐
Heavy	☐	☐	☐	☐	☐	☐	☐	☐	☐	☐
Ultra	☐	☐	☐	☐	☐	☐	☐	☐	☐	☐
PAIN 1	☐	☐	☐	☐	☐	☐	☐	☐	☐	☐
2	☐	☐	☐	☐	☐	☐	☐	☐	☐	☐
3	☐	☐	☐	☐	☐	☐	☐	☐	☐	☐
4	☐	☐	☐	☐	☐	☐	☐	☐	☐	☐
5	☐	☐	☐	☐	☐	☐	☐	☐	☐	☐

Period Symptoms

Discomfort: ☐ Cramps ☐ Mood Swings ☐ Headache ☐ Hunger
☐ Tender Breasts ☐ Back Pain ☐ Fatigue ☐ Acne ☐ Sleep Issues

Digestion: ☐ Nausea ☐ Ache ☐ Bloat ☐ Diarrhea ☐ Constipation

Cravings: ☐ Sweet ☐ Spice ☐ Salt ☐ Carb ☐ Cheese ☐ Alcohol

Emotions: ☐ Happy ☐ Energetic ☐ Motivated ☐ Calm ☐ Angry
☐ Irritated ☐ Sad ☐ Stressed ☐ Anxious ☐ Excited ☐ In Love

Body Check   *Weight:* _____

Exercise: ☐ Stretches ☐ Yoga ☐ Cardio ☐ Weights ☐ Impact

Diet: ☐ Healthy Eating ☐ Standard Diet ☐ Processed Food

Discharge Normal Colors: ☐ Clear ☐ White ☐ Pink ☐ Brown
NOT Normal: ☐ Yellow ☐ Green ☐ Gray ☐ White Lumps

Problems: ☐ Itchy ☐ Burning ☐ Soreness ☐ Weird Discharge
☐ Funky Smell ☐ Odd Changes ☐ Pain with Peeing ☐ Pain with Sex

Sex: ☐ Nope ☐ Solo ☐ Girls Only ☐ Protected ☐ Unprotected

Birth Control: ☐ Condom ☐ IUD ☐ Pill ☐ Patch ☐ Implant
☐ Shot ☐ Vaginal Ring ☐ Tubal Ligation ☐ Partner Vasectomy

Notes

_____

_____

_____

_____

_____

_____

My Period   *Month:_____   Year:_____*

	SUN	MON	TUE	WED	THU	FRI	SAT
Start							
End							
Day Length							
Next Period Expected							

Start

End

Day Length

Next Period Expected

Arrived:

☐ On Time ☐ Early ☐ Late

Feels:

☐ Normal ☐ See Doc

FLOW	1	2	3	4	5	6	7	8	9	10
Spotting	☐	☐	☐	☐	☐	☐	☐	☐	☐	☐
Light	☐	☐	☐	☐	☐	☐	☐	☐	☐	☐
Medium	☐	☐	☐	☐	☐	☐	☐	☐	☐	☐
Heavy	☐	☐	☐	☐	☐	☐	☐	☐	☐	☐
Ultra	☐	☐	☐	☐	☐	☐	☐	☐	☐	☐
PAIN 1	☐	☐	☐	☐	☐	☐	☐	☐	☐	☐
2	☐	☐	☐	☐	☐	☐	☐	☐	☐	☐
3	☐	☐	☐	☐	☐	☐	☐	☐	☐	☐
4	☐	☐	☐	☐	☐	☐	☐	☐	☐	☐
5	☐	☐	☐	☐	☐	☐	☐	☐	☐	☐

Period Symptoms

Discomfort: ☐ Cramps ☐ Mood Swings ☐ Headache ☐ Hunger
☐ Tender Breasts ☐ Back Pain ☐ Fatigue ☐ Acne ☐ Sleep Issues

Digestion: ☐ Nausea ☐ Ache ☐ Bloat ☐ Diarrhea ☐ Constipation

Cravings: ☐ Sweet ☐ Spice ☐ Salt ☐ Carb ☐ Cheese ☐ Alcohol

Emotions: ☐ Happy ☐ Energetic ☐ Motivated ☐ Calm ☐ Angry
☐ Irritated ☐ Sad ☐ Stressed ☐ Anxious ☐ Excited ☐ In Love

Body Check   Weight: _____

Exercise: ☐ Stretches ☐ Yoga ☐ Cardio ☐ Weights ☐ Impact

Diet: ☐ Healthy Eating ☐ Standard Diet ☐ Processed Food

Discharge Normal Colors: ☐ Clear ☐ White ☐ Pink ☐ Brown
   NOT Normal: ☐ Yellow ☐ Green ☐ Gray ☐ White Lumps

Problems: ☐ Itchy ☐ Burning ☐ Soreness ☐ Weird Discharge
☐ Funky Smell ☐ Odd Changes ☐ Pain with Peeing ☐ Pain with Sex

Sex: ☐ Nope ☐ Solo ☐ Girls Only ☐ Protected ☐ Unprotected

Birth Control: ☐ Condom ☐ IUD ☐ Pill ☐ Patch ☐ Implant
☐ Shot ☐ Vaginal Ring ☐ Tubal Ligation ☐ Partner Vasectomy

Notes

_____

_____

_____

_____

_____

_____

My Period Month:_____ Year:_____

	SUN	MON	TUE	WED	THU	FRI	SAT
Start							
End							
Day Length							
Next Period Expected							

Arrived:

☐ On Time ☐ Early ☐ Late

Feels:

☐ Normal ☐ See Doc

FLOW	1	2	3	4	5	6	7	8	9	10
Spotting	☐	☐	☐	☐	☐	☐	☐	☐	☐	☐
Light	☐	☐	☐	☐	☐	☐	☐	☐	☐	☐
Medium	☐	☐	☐	☐	☐	☐	☐	☐	☐	☐
Heavy	☐	☐	☐	☐	☐	☐	☐	☐	☐	☐
Ultra	☐	☐	☐	☐	☐	☐	☐	☐	☐	☐
PAIN 1	☐	☐	☐	☐	☐	☐	☐	☐	☐	☐
2	☐	☐	☐	☐	☐	☐	☐	☐	☐	☐
3	☐	☐	☐	☐	☐	☐	☐	☐	☐	☐
4	☐	☐	☐	☐	☐	☐	☐	☐	☐	☐
5	☐	☐	☐	☐	☐	☐	☐	☐	☐	☐

Period Symptoms

Discomfort: ☐ Cramps ☐ Mood Swings ☐ Headache ☐ Hunger ☐ Tender Breasts ☐ Back Pain ☐ Fatigue ☐ Acne ☐ Sleep Issues

Digestion: ☐ Nausea ☐ Ache ☐ Bloat ☐ Diarrhea ☐ Constipation

Cravings: ☐ Sweet ☐ Spice ☐ Salt ☐ Carb ☐ Cheese ☐ Alcohol

Emotions: ☐ Happy ☐ Energetic ☐ Motivated ☐ Calm ☐ Angry ☐ Irritated ☐ Sad ☐ Stressed ☐ Anxious ☐ Excited ☐ In Love

Body Check   *Weight:* _____

Exercise: ☐ Stretches ☐ Yoga ☐ Cardio ☐ Weights ☐ Impact

Diet: ☐ Healthy Eating ☐ Standard Diet ☐ Processed Food

Discharge Normal Colors: ☐ Clear ☐ White ☐ Pink ☐ Brown
   NOT Normal: ☐ Yellow ☐ Green ☐ Gray ☐ White Lumps

Problems: ☐ Itchy ☐ Burning ☐ Soreness ☐ Weird Discharge ☐ Funky Smell ☐ Odd Changes ☐ Pain with Peeing ☐ Pain with Sex

Sex: ☐ Nope ☐ Solo ☐ Girls Only ☐ Protected ☐ Unprotected

Birth Control: ☐ Condom ☐ IUD ☐ Pill ☐ Patch ☐ Implant ☐ Shot ☐ Vaginal Ring ☐ Tubal Ligation ☐ Partner Vasectomy

Notes

_____

_____

_____

_____

_____

_____

My Period

*Month:*_____ *Year:*_____

Start		*SUN*	*MON*	*TUE*	*WED*	*THU*	*FRI*	*SAT*

Start

[ ]

End

[ ]

Day Length

[ ]

Next Period Expected

[ ]

Arrived:

☐ On Time ☐ Early ☐ Late

Feels:

☐ Normal ☐ See Doc

FLOW	1	2	3	4	5	6	7	8	9	10
Spotting	☐	☐	☐	☐	☐	☐	☐	☐	☐	☐
Light	☐	☐	☐	☐	☐	☐	☐	☐	☐	☐
Medium	☐	☐	☐	☐	☐	☐	☐	☐	☐	☐
Heavy	☐	☐	☐	☐	☐	☐	☐	☐	☐	☐
Ultra	☐	☐	☐	☐	☐	☐	☐	☐	☐	☐
PAIN 1	☐	☐	☐	☐	☐	☐	☐	☐	☐	☐
2	☐	☐	☐	☐	☐	☐	☐	☐	☐	☐
3	☐	☐	☐	☐	☐	☐	☐	☐	☐	☐
4	☐	☐	☐	☐	☐	☐	☐	☐	☐	☐
5	☐	☐	☐	☐	☐	☐	☐	☐	☐	☐

Period Symptoms

Discomfort: ☐ Cramps ☐ Mood Swings ☐ Headache ☐ Hunger
☐ Tender Breasts ☐ Back Pain ☐ Fatigue ☐ Acne ☐ Sleep Issues

Digestion: ☐ Nausea ☐ Ache ☐ Bloat ☐ Diarrhea ☐ Constipation

Cravings: ☐ Sweet ☐ Spice ☐ Salt ☐ Carb ☐ Cheese ☐ Alcohol

Emotions: ☐ Happy ☐ Energetic ☐ Motivated ☐ Calm ☐ Angry
☐ Irritated ☐ Sad ☐ Stressed ☐ Anxious ☐ Excited ☐ In Love

Body Check   *Weight:* _____

Exercise: ☐ Stretches ☐ Yoga ☐ Cardio ☐ Weights ☐ Impact

Diet: ☐ Healthy Eating ☐ Standard Diet ☐ Processed Food

Discharge Normal Colors: ☐ Clear ☐ White ☐ Pink ☐ Brown
  NOT Normal: ☐ Yellow ☐ Green ☐ Gray ☐ White Lumps

Problems: ☐ Itchy ☐ Burning ☐ Soreness ☐ Weird Discharge
☐ Funky Smell ☐ Odd Changes ☐ Pain with Peeing ☐ Pain with Sex

Sex: ☐ Nope ☐ Solo ☐ Girls Only ☐ Protected ☐ Unprotected

Birth Control: ☐ Condom ☐ IUD ☐ Pill ☐ Patch ☐ Implant
☐ Shot ☐ Vaginal Ring ☐ Tubal Ligation ☐ Partner Vasectomy

Notes

_____

_____

_____

_____

_____

_____

My Period   *Month:_____   Year:_____*

Start	**SUN**	**MON**	**TUE**	**WED**	**THU**	**FRI**	**SAT**
End							
Day Length							
Next Period Expected							

Arrived:

☐ On Time ☐ Early ☐ Late

Feels:

☐ Normal ☐ See Doc

FLOW	1	2	3	4	5	6	7	8	9	10
Spotting	☐	☐	☐	☐	☐	☐	☐	☐	☐	☐
Light	☐	☐	☐	☐	☐	☐	☐	☐	☐	☐
Medium	☐	☐	☐	☐	☐	☐	☐	☐	☐	☐
Heavy	☐	☐	☐	☐	☐	☐	☐	☐	☐	☐
Ultra	☐	☐	☐	☐	☐	☐	☐	☐	☐	☐
PAIN 1	☐	☐	☐	☐	☐	☐	☐	☐	☐	☐
2	☐	☐	☐	☐	☐	☐	☐	☐	☐	☐
3	☐	☐	☐	☐	☐	☐	☐	☐	☐	☐
4	☐	☐	☐	☐	☐	☐	☐	☐	☐	☐
5	☐	☐	☐	☐	☐	☐	☐	☐	☐	☐

Period Symptoms

Discomfort: ☐ Cramps ☐ Mood Swings ☐ Headache ☐ Hunger
☐ Tender Breasts ☐ Back Pain ☐ Fatigue ☐ Acne ☐ Sleep Issues

Digestion: ☐ Nausea ☐ Ache ☐ Bloat ☐ Diarrhea ☐ Constipation

Cravings: ☐ Sweet ☐ Spice ☐ Salt ☐ Carb ☐ Cheese ☐ Alcohol

Emotions: ☐ Happy ☐ Energetic ☐ Motivated ☐ Calm ☐ Angry
☐ Irritated ☐ Sad ☐ Stressed ☐ Anxious ☐ Excited ☐ In Love

Body Check   Weight: _____

Exercise: ☐ Stretches ☐ Yoga ☐ Cardio ☐ Weights ☐ Impact

Diet: ☐ Healthy Eating ☐ Standard Diet ☐ Processed Food

Discharge Normal Colors: ☐ Clear ☐ White ☐ Pink ☐ Brown
  NOT Normal: ☐ Yellow ☐ Green ☐ Gray ☐ White Lumps

Problems: ☐ Itchy ☐ Burning ☐ Soreness ☐ Weird Discharge
☐ Funky Smell ☐ Odd Changes ☐ Pain with Peeing ☐ Pain with Sex

Sex: ☐ Nope ☐ Solo ☐ Girls Only ☐ Protected ☐ Unprotected

Birth Control: ☐ Condom ☐ IUD ☐ Pill ☐ Patch ☐ Implant
☐ Shot ☐ Vaginal Ring ☐ Tubal Ligation ☐ Partner Vasectomy

Notes

_____

_____

_____

_____

_____

_____

My Period Month:_____ Year:_____

	Start		SUN	MON	TUE	WED	THU	FRI	SAT

Start
[ ]

End
[ ]

Day Length
[ ]

Next Period Expected
[ ]

Arrived:

☐ On Time ☐ Early ☐ Late

Feels:

☐ Normal ☐ See Doc

FLOW	1	2	3	4	5	6	7	8	9	10
Spotting	☐	☐	☐	☐	☐	☐	☐	☐	☐	☐
Light	☐	☐	☐	☐	☐	☐	☐	☐	☐	☐
Medium	☐	☐	☐	☐	☐	☐	☐	☐	☐	☐
Heavy	☐	☐	☐	☐	☐	☐	☐	☐	☐	☐
Ultra	☐	☐	☐	☐	☐	☐	☐	☐	☐	☐
PAIN 1	☐	☐	☐	☐	☐	☐	☐	☐	☐	☐
2	☐	☐	☐	☐	☐	☐	☐	☐	☐	☐
3	☐	☐	☐	☐	☐	☐	☐	☐	☐	☐
4	☐	☐	☐	☐	☐	☐	☐	☐	☐	☐
5	☐	☐	☐	☐	☐	☐	☐	☐	☐	☐

Period Symptoms

Discomfort: ☐ Cramps ☐ Mood Swings ☐ Headache ☐ Hunger
☐ Tender Breasts ☐ Back Pain ☐ Fatigue ☐ Acne ☐ Sleep Issues

Digestion: ☐ Nausea ☐ Ache ☐ Bloat ☐ Diarrhea ☐ Constipation

Cravings: ☐ Sweet ☐ Spice ☐ Salt ☐ Carb ☐ Cheese ☐ Alcohol

Emotions: ☐ Happy ☐ Energetic ☐ Motivated ☐ Calm ☐ Angry
☐ Irritated ☐ Sad ☐ Stressed ☐ Anxious ☐ Excited ☐ In Love

Body Check   *Weight:* _____

Exercise: ☐ Stretches ☐ Yoga ☐ Cardio ☐ Weights ☐ Impact

Diet: ☐ Healthy Eating ☐ Standard Diet ☐ Processed Food

Discharge Normal Colors: ☐ Clear ☐ White ☐ Pink ☐ Brown
NOT Normal: ☐ Yellow ☐ Green ☐ Gray ☐ White Lumps

Problems: ☐ Itchy ☐ Burning ☐ Soreness ☐ Weird Discharge
☐ Funky Smell ☐ Odd Changes ☐ Pain with Peeing ☐ Pain with Sex

Sex: ☐ Nope ☐ Solo ☐ Girls Only ☐ Protected ☐ Unprotected

Birth Control: ☐ Condom ☐ IUD ☐ Pill ☐ Patch ☐ Implant
☐ Shot ☐ Vaginal Ring ☐ Tubal Ligation ☐ Partner Vasectomy

Notes

_____

_____

_____

_____

_____

_____

My Period   *Month:_____*   *Year:_____*

Start	SUN	MON	TUE	WED	THU	FRI	SAT

End

Day Length

Next Period Expected

Arrived:

☐ On Time ☐ Early ☐ Late

Feels:

☐ Normal ☐ See Doc

FLOW	1	2	3	4	5	6	7	8	9	10
Spotting	☐	☐	☐	☐	☐	☐	☐	☐	☐	☐
Light	☐	☐	☐	☐	☐	☐	☐	☐	☐	☐
Medium	☐	☐	☐	☐	☐	☐	☐	☐	☐	☐
Heavy	☐	☐	☐	☐	☐	☐	☐	☐	☐	☐
Ultra	☐	☐	☐	☐	☐	☐	☐	☐	☐	☐
PAIN 1	☐	☐	☐	☐	☐	☐	☐	☐	☐	☐
2	☐	☐	☐	☐	☐	☐	☐	☐	☐	☐
3	☐	☐	☐	☐	☐	☐	☐	☐	☐	☐
4	☐	☐	☐	☐	☐	☐	☐	☐	☐	☐
5	☐	☐	☐	☐	☐	☐	☐	☐	☐	☐

Period Symptoms

Discomfort: ☐ Cramps ☐ Mood Swings ☐ Headache ☐ Hunger
☐ Tender Breasts ☐ Back Pain ☐ Fatigue ☐ Acne ☐ Sleep Issues

Digestion: ☐ Nausea ☐ Ache ☐ Bloat ☐ Diarrhea ☐ Constipation

Cravings: ☐ Sweet ☐ Spice ☐ Salt ☐ Carb ☐ Cheese ☐ Alcohol

Emotions: ☐ Happy ☐ Energetic ☐ Motivated ☐ Calm ☐ Angry
☐ Irritated ☐ Sad ☐ Stressed ☐ Anxious ☐ Excited ☐ In Love

Body Check

Weight: _____

Exercise: ☐ Stretches ☐ Yoga ☐ Cardio ☐ Weights ☐ Impact

Diet: ☐ Healthy Eating ☐ Standard Diet ☐ Processed Food

Discharge Normal Colors: ☐ Clear ☐ White ☐ Pink ☐ Brown
NOT Normal: ☐ Yellow ☐ Green ☐ Gray ☐ White Lumps

Problems: ☐ Itchy ☐ Burning ☐ Soreness ☐ Weird Discharge
☐ Funky Smell ☐ Odd Changes ☐ Pain with Peeing ☐ Pain with Sex

Sex: ☐ Nope ☐ Solo ☐ Girls Only ☐ Protected ☐ Unprotected

Birth Control: ☐ Condom ☐ IUD ☐ Pill ☐ Patch ☐ Implant
☐ Shot ☐ Vaginal Ring ☐ Tubal Ligation ☐ Partner Vasectomy

Notes

_____

_____

_____

_____

_____

_____

My Period *Month:_____* *Year:_____*

Start	SUN	MON	TUE	WED	THU	FRI	SAT

End

Day Length

Next Period Expected

Arrived:

☐ On Time ☐ Early ☐ Late

Feels:

☐ Normal ☐ See Doc

FLOW	1	2	3	4	5	6	7	8	9	10
Spotting	☐	☐	☐	☐	☐	☐	☐	☐	☐	☐
Light	☐	☐	☐	☐	☐	☐	☐	☐	☐	☐
Medium	☐	☐	☐	☐	☐	☐	☐	☐	☐	☐
Heavy	☐	☐	☐	☐	☐	☐	☐	☐	☐	☐
Ultra	☐	☐	☐	☐	☐	☐	☐	☐	☐	☐
PAIN 1	☐	☐	☐	☐	☐	☐	☐	☐	☐	☐
2	☐	☐	☐	☐	☐	☐	☐	☐	☐	☐
3	☐	☐	☐	☐	☐	☐	☐	☐	☐	☐
4	☐	☐	☐	☐	☐	☐	☐	☐	☐	☐
5	☐	☐	☐	☐	☐	☐	☐	☐	☐	☐

Period Symptoms

Discomfort: ☐ Cramps ☐ Mood Swings ☐ Headache ☐ Hunger
☐ Tender Breasts ☐ Back Pain ☐ Fatigue ☐ Acne ☐ Sleep Issues

Digestion: ☐ Nausea ☐ Ache ☐ Bloat ☐ Diarrhea ☐ Constipation

Cravings: ☐ Sweet ☐ Spice ☐ Salt ☐ Carb ☐ Cheese ☐ Alcohol

Emotions: ☐ Happy ☐ Energetic ☐ Motivated ☐ Calm ☐ Angry
☐ Irritated ☐ Sad ☐ Stressed ☐ Anxious ☐ Excited ☐ In Love

Body Check   *Weight:* _____

Exercise: ☐ Stretches ☐ Yoga ☐ Cardio ☐ Weights ☐ Impact

Diet: ☐ Healthy Eating ☐ Standard Diet ☐ Processed Food

Discharge Normal Colors: ☐ Clear ☐ White ☐ Pink ☐ Brown
   NOT Normal: ☐ Yellow ☐ Green ☐ Gray ☐ White Lumps

Problems: ☐ Itchy ☐ Burning ☐ Soreness ☐ Weird Discharge
☐ Funky Smell ☐ Odd Changes ☐ Pain with Peeing ☐ Pain with Sex

Sex: ☐ Nope ☐ Solo ☐ Girls Only ☐ Protected ☐ Unprotected

Birth Control: ☐ Condom ☐ IUD ☐ Pill ☐ Patch ☐ Implant
☐ Shot ☐ Vaginal Ring ☐ Tubal Ligation ☐ Partner Vasectomy

Notes

_____

_____

_____

_____

_____

_____

My Period   *Month:_____   Year:_____*

Start	SUN	MON	TUE	WED	THU	FRI	SAT

End

Day Length

Next Period Expected

Arrived:

☐ On Time ☐ Early ☐ Late

Feels:

☐ Normal ☐ See Doc

FLOW	1	2	3	4	5	6	7	8	9	10
Spotting	☐	☐	☐	☐	☐	☐	☐	☐	☐	☐
Light	☐	☐	☐	☐	☐	☐	☐	☐	☐	☐
Medium	☐	☐	☐	☐	☐	☐	☐	☐	☐	☐
Heavy	☐	☐	☐	☐	☐	☐	☐	☐	☐	☐
Ultra	☐	☐	☐	☐	☐	☐	☐	☐	☐	☐
PAIN 1	☐	☐	☐	☐	☐	☐	☐	☐	☐	☐
2	☐	☐	☐	☐	☐	☐	☐	☐	☐	☐
3	☐	☐	☐	☐	☐	☐	☐	☐	☐	☐
4	☐	☐	☐	☐	☐	☐	☐	☐	☐	☐
5	☐	☐	☐	☐	☐	☐	☐	☐	☐	☐

Period Symptoms

Discomfort: ☐ Cramps ☐ Mood Swings ☐ Headache ☐ Hunger
☐ Tender Breasts ☐ Back Pain ☐ Fatigue ☐ Acne ☐ Sleep Issues

Digestion: ☐ Nausea ☐ Ache ☐ Bloat ☐ Diarrhea ☐ Constipation

Cravings: ☐ Sweet ☐ Spice ☐ Salt ☐ Carb ☐ Cheese ☐ Alcohol

Emotions: ☐ Happy ☐ Energetic ☐ Motivated ☐ Calm ☐ Angry
☐ Irritated ☐ Sad ☐ Stressed ☐ Anxious ☐ Excited ☐ In Love

Body Check   *Weight:* _____

Exercise: ☐ Stretches ☐ Yoga ☐ Cardio ☐ Weights ☐ Impact

Diet: ☐ Healthy Eating ☐ Standard Diet ☐ Processed Food

Discharge Normal Colors: ☐ Clear ☐ White ☐ Pink ☐ Brown
   NOT Normal: ☐ Yellow ☐ Green ☐ Gray ☐ White Lumps

Problems: ☐ Itchy ☐ Burning ☐ Soreness ☐ Weird Discharge
☐ Funky Smell ☐ Odd Changes ☐ Pain with Peeing ☐ Pain with Sex

Sex: ☐ Nope ☐ Solo ☐ Girls Only ☐ Protected ☐ Unprotected

Birth Control: ☐ Condom ☐ IUD ☐ Pill ☐ Patch ☐ Implant
☐ Shot ☐ Vaginal Ring ☐ Tubal Ligation ☐ Partner Vasectomy

Notes

_____

_____

_____

_____

_____

_____

My Period   *Month:_____   Year:_____*

Start	*SUN*	*MON*	*TUE*	*WED*	*THU*	*FRI*	*SAT*
End							
Day Length							
Next Period Expected							

Arrived:

☐ On Time ☐ Early ☐ Late

Feels:

☐ Normal ☐ See Doc

FLOW	1	2	3	4	5	6	7	8	9	10
Spotting	☐	☐	☐	☐	☐	☐	☐	☐	☐	☐
Light	☐	☐	☐	☐	☐	☐	☐	☐	☐	☐
Medium	☐	☐	☐	☐	☐	☐	☐	☐	☐	☐
Heavy	☐	☐	☐	☐	☐	☐	☐	☐	☐	☐
Ultra	☐	☐	☐	☐	☐	☐	☐	☐	☐	☐
PAIN 1	☐	☐	☐	☐	☐	☐	☐	☐	☐	☐
2	☐	☐	☐	☐	☐	☐	☐	☐	☐	☐
3	☐	☐	☐	☐	☐	☐	☐	☐	☐	☐
4	☐	☐	☐	☐	☐	☐	☐	☐	☐	☐
5	☐	☐	☐	☐	☐	☐	☐	☐	☐	☐

Period Symptoms

Discomfort: ☐ Cramps ☐ Mood Swings ☐ Headache ☐ Hunger
☐ Tender Breasts ☐ Back Pain ☐ Fatigue ☐ Acne ☐ Sleep Issues

Digestion: ☐ Nausea ☐ Ache ☐ Bloat ☐ Diarrhea ☐ Constipation

Cravings: ☐ Sweet ☐ Spice ☐ Salt ☐ Carb ☐ Cheese ☐ Alcohol

Emotions: ☐ Happy ☐ Energetic ☐ Motivated ☐ Calm ☐ Angry
☐ Irritated ☐ Sad ☐ Stressed ☐ Anxious ☐ Excited ☐ In Love

Body Check   *Weight:* _____

Exercise: ☐ Stretches ☐ Yoga ☐ Cardio ☐ Weights ☐ Impact

Diet: ☐ Healthy Eating ☐ Standard Diet ☐ Processed Food

Discharge Normal Colors: ☐ Clear ☐ White ☐ Pink ☐ Brown
NOT Normal: ☐ Yellow ☐ Green ☐ Gray ☐ White Lumps

Problems: ☐ Itchy ☐ Burning ☐ Soreness ☐ Weird Discharge
☐ Funky Smell ☐ Odd Changes ☐ Pain with Peeing ☐ Pain with Sex

Sex: ☐ Nope ☐ Solo ☐ Girls Only ☐ Protected ☐ Unprotected

Birth Control: ☐ Condom ☐ IUD ☐ Pill ☐ Patch ☐ Implant
☐ Shot ☐ Vaginal Ring ☐ Tubal Ligation ☐ Partner Vasectomy

Notes

_____

_____

_____

_____

_____

_____

My Period   *Month:_____*   *Year:_____*

Start	*SUN*	*MON*	*TUE*	*WED*	*THU*	*FRI*	*SAT*
End							
Day Length							
Next Period Expected							

Arrived:

☐ On Time ☐ Early ☐ Late

Feels:

☐ Normal ☐ See Doc

FLOW	1	2	3	4	5	6	7	8	9	10
Spotting	☐	☐	☐	☐	☐	☐	☐	☐	☐	☐
Light	☐	☐	☐	☐	☐	☐	☐	☐	☐	☐
Medium	☐	☐	☐	☐	☐	☐	☐	☐	☐	☐
Heavy	☐	☐	☐	☐	☐	☐	☐	☐	☐	☐
Ultra	☐	☐	☐	☐	☐	☐	☐	☐	☐	☐
PAIN 1	☐	☐	☐	☐	☐	☐	☐	☐	☐	☐
2	☐	☐	☐	☐	☐	☐	☐	☐	☐	☐
3	☐	☐	☐	☐	☐	☐	☐	☐	☐	☐
4	☐	☐	☐	☐	☐	☐	☐	☐	☐	☐
5	☐	☐	☐	☐	☐	☐	☐	☐	☐	☐

Period Symptoms

Discomfort: ☐ Cramps ☐ Mood Swings ☐ Headache ☐ Hunger
☐ Tender Breasts ☐ Back Pain ☐ Fatigue ☐ Acne ☐ Sleep Issues

Digestion: ☐ Nausea ☐ Ache ☐ Bloat ☐ Diarrhea ☐ Constipation

Cravings: ☐ Sweet ☐ Spice ☐ Salt ☐ Carb ☐ Cheese ☐ Alcohol

Emotions: ☐ Happy ☐ Energetic ☐ Motivated ☐ Calm ☐ Angry
☐ Irritated ☐ Sad ☐ Stressed ☐ Anxious ☐ Excited ☐ In Love

Body Check   *Weight:* _____

Exercise: ☐ Stretches ☐ Yoga ☐ Cardio ☐ Weights ☐ Impact

Diet: ☐ Healthy Eating ☐ Standard Diet ☐ Processed Food

Discharge Normal Colors: ☐ Clear ☐ White ☐ Pink ☐ Brown
NOT Normal: ☐ Yellow ☐ Green ☐ Gray ☐ White Lumps

Problems: ☐ Itchy ☐ Burning ☐ Soreness ☐ Weird Discharge
☐ Funky Smell ☐ Odd Changes ☐ Pain with Peeing ☐ Pain with Sex

Sex: ☐ Nope ☐ Solo ☐ Girls Only ☐ Protected ☐ Unprotected

Birth Control: ☐ Condom ☐ IUD ☐ Pill ☐ Patch ☐ Implant
☐ Shot ☐ Vaginal Ring ☐ Tubal Ligation ☐ Partner Vasectomy

Notes

_____

_____

_____

_____

_____

_____

My Period   *Month:*_____   *Year:*_____

Start	*SUN*	*MON*	*TUE*	*WED*	*THU*	*FRI*	*SAT*

End

Day Length

Next Period Expected

Arrived:

☐ On Time ☐ Early ☐ Late

Feels:

☐ Normal ☐ See Doc

FLOW	1	2	3	4	5	6	7	8	9	10
Spotting	☐	☐	☐	☐	☐	☐	☐	☐	☐	☐
Light	☐	☐	☐	☐	☐	☐	☐	☐	☐	☐
Medium	☐	☐	☐	☐	☐	☐	☐	☐	☐	☐
Heavy	☐	☐	☐	☐	☐	☐	☐	☐	☐	☐
Ultra	☐	☐	☐	☐	☐	☐	☐	☐	☐	☐
PAIN 1	☐	☐	☐	☐	☐	☐	☐	☐	☐	☐
2	☐	☐	☐	☐	☐	☐	☐	☐	☐	☐
3	☐	☐	☐	☐	☐	☐	☐	☐	☐	☐
4	☐	☐	☐	☐	☐	☐	☐	☐	☐	☐
5	☐	☐	☐	☐	☐	☐	☐	☐	☐	☐

Period Symptoms

Discomfort: ☐ Cramps ☐ Mood Swings ☐ Headache ☐ Hunger
☐ Tender Breasts ☐ Back Pain ☐ Fatigue ☐ Acne ☐ Sleep Issues

Digestion: ☐ Nausea ☐ Ache ☐ Bloat ☐ Diarrhea ☐ Constipation

Cravings: ☐ Sweet ☐ Spice ☐ Salt ☐ Carb ☐ Cheese ☐ Alcohol

Emotions: ☐ Happy ☐ Energetic ☐ Motivated ☐ Calm ☐ Angry
☐ Irritated ☐ Sad ☐ Stressed ☐ Anxious ☐ Excited ☐ In Love

Body Check   Weight: _____

Exercise: ☐ Stretches ☐ Yoga ☐ Cardio ☐ Weights ☐ Impact

Diet: ☐ Healthy Eating ☐ Standard Diet ☐ Processed Food

Discharge Normal Colors: ☐ Clear ☐ White ☐ Pink ☐ Brown
NOT Normal: ☐ Yellow ☐ Green ☐ Gray ☐ White Lumps

Problems: ☐ Itchy ☐ Burning ☐ Soreness ☐ Weird Discharge
☐ Funky Smell ☐ Odd Changes ☐ Pain with Peeing ☐ Pain with Sex

Sex: ☐ Nope ☐ Solo ☐ Girls Only ☐ Protected ☐ Unprotected

Birth Control: ☐ Condom ☐ IUD ☐ Pill ☐ Patch ☐ Implant
☐ Shot ☐ Vaginal Ring ☐ Tubal Ligation ☐ Partner Vasectomy

Notes

_____

_____

_____

_____

_____

_____

My Period *Month:_____* *Year:_____*

Start

	SUN	MON	TUE	WED	THU	FRI	SAT

End

Day Length

Next Period Expected

Arrived:

☐ On Time ☐ Early ☐ Late

Feels:

☐ Normal ☐ See Doc

FLOW	1	2	3	4	5	6	7	8	9	10
Spotting	☐	☐	☐	☐	☐	☐	☐	☐	☐	☐
Light	☐	☐	☐	☐	☐	☐	☐	☐	☐	☐
Medium	☐	☐	☐	☐	☐	☐	☐	☐	☐	☐
Heavy	☐	☐	☐	☐	☐	☐	☐	☐	☐	☐
Ultra	☐	☐	☐	☐	☐	☐	☐	☐	☐	☐
PAIN 1	☐	☐	☐	☐	☐	☐	☐	☐	☐	☐
2	☐	☐	☐	☐	☐	☐	☐	☐	☐	☐
3	☐	☐	☐	☐	☐	☐	☐	☐	☐	☐
4	☐	☐	☐	☐	☐	☐	☐	☐	☐	☐
5	☐	☐	☐	☐	☐	☐	☐	☐	☐	☐

Period Symptoms

Discomfort: ☐ Cramps ☐ Mood Swings ☐ Headache ☐ Hunger
☐ Tender Breasts ☐ Back Pain ☐ Fatigue ☐ Acne ☐ Sleep Issues

Digestion: ☐ Nausea ☐ Ache ☐ Bloat ☐ Diarrhea ☐ Constipation

Cravings: ☐ Sweet ☐ Spice ☐ Salt ☐ Carb ☐ Cheese ☐ Alcohol

Emotions: ☐ Happy ☐ Energetic ☐ Motivated ☐ Calm ☐ Angry
☐ Irritated ☐ Sad ☐ Stressed ☐ Anxious ☐ Excited ☐ In Love

Body Check   Weight: _____

Exercise: ☐ Stretches ☐ Yoga ☐ Cardio ☐ Weights ☐ Impact

Diet: ☐ Healthy Eating ☐ Standard Diet ☐ Processed Food

Discharge Normal Colors: ☐ Clear ☐ White ☐ Pink ☐ Brown
   NOT Normal: ☐ Yellow ☐ Green ☐ Gray ☐ White Lumps

Problems: ☐ Itchy ☐ Burning ☐ Soreness ☐ Weird Discharge
☐ Funky Smell ☐ Odd Changes ☐ Pain with Peeing ☐ Pain with Sex

Sex: ☐ Nope ☐ Solo ☐ Girls Only ☐ Protected ☐ Unprotected

Birth Control: ☐ Condom ☐ IUD ☐ Pill ☐ Patch ☐ Implant
☐ Shot ☐ Vaginal Ring ☐ Tubal Ligation ☐ Partner Vasectomy

Notes

_____

_____

_____

_____

_____

_____

My Period   *Month:_____   Year:_____*

Start

End

Day Length

Next Period Expected

SUN	MON	TUE	WED	THU	FRI	SAT

Arrived:

☐ On Time ☐ Early ☐ Late

Feels:

☐ Normal ☐ See Doc

FLOW	1	2	3	4	5	6	7	8	9	10
Spotting	☐	☐	☐	☐	☐	☐	☐	☐	☐	☐
Light	☐	☐	☐	☐	☐	☐	☐	☐	☐	☐
Medium	☐	☐	☐	☐	☐	☐	☐	☐	☐	☐
Heavy	☐	☐	☐	☐	☐	☐	☐	☐	☐	☐
Ultra	☐	☐	☐	☐	☐	☐	☐	☐	☐	☐
PAIN 1	☐	☐	☐	☐	☐	☐	☐	☐	☐	☐
2	☐	☐	☐	☐	☐	☐	☐	☐	☐	☐
3	☐	☐	☐	☐	☐	☐	☐	☐	☐	☐
4	☐	☐	☐	☐	☐	☐	☐	☐	☐	☐
5	☐	☐	☐	☐	☐	☐	☐	☐	☐	☐

Period Symptoms

Discomfort: ☐ Cramps ☐ Mood Swings ☐ Headache ☐ Hunger
☐ Tender Breasts ☐ Back Pain ☐ Fatigue ☐ Acne ☐ Sleep Issues

Digestion: ☐ Nausea ☐ Ache ☐ Bloat ☐ Diarrhea ☐ Constipation

Cravings: ☐ Sweet ☐ Spice ☐ Salt ☐ Carb ☐ Cheese ☐ Alcohol

Emotions: ☐ Happy ☐ Energetic ☐ Motivated ☐ Calm ☐ Angry
☐ Irritated ☐ Sad ☐ Stressed ☐ Anxious ☐ Excited ☐ In Love

Body Check   *Weight:* _____

Exercise: ☐ Stretches ☐ Yoga ☐ Cardio ☐ Weights ☐ Impact

Diet: ☐ Healthy Eating ☐ Standard Diet ☐ Processed Food

Discharge Normal Colors: ☐ Clear ☐ White ☐ Pink ☐ Brown
NOT Normal: ☐ Yellow ☐ Green ☐ Gray ☐ White Lumps

Problems: ☐ Itchy ☐ Burning ☐ Soreness ☐ Weird Discharge
☐ Funky Smell ☐ Odd Changes ☐ Pain with Peeing ☐ Pain with Sex

Sex: ☐ Nope ☐ Solo ☐ Girls Only ☐ Protected ☐ Unprotected

Birth Control: ☐ Condom ☐ IUD ☐ Pill ☐ Patch ☐ Implant
☐ Shot ☐ Vaginal Ring ☐ Tubal Ligation ☐ Partner Vasectomy

Notes

_____

_____

_____

_____

_____

_____

My Period   *Month:_____*   *Year:_____*

Start

SUN	MON	TUE	WED	THU	FRI	SAT

End

Day Length

Next Period Expected

Arrived:

☐ On Time ☐ Early ☐ Late

Feels:

☐ Normal ☐ See Doc

FLOW	1	2	3	4	5	6	7	8	9	10
Spotting	☐	☐	☐	☐	☐	☐	☐	☐	☐	☐
Light	☐	☐	☐	☐	☐	☐	☐	☐	☐	☐
Medium	☐	☐	☐	☐	☐	☐	☐	☐	☐	☐
Heavy	☐	☐	☐	☐	☐	☐	☐	☐	☐	☐
Ultra	☐	☐	☐	☐	☐	☐	☐	☐	☐	☐
PAIN 1	☐	☐	☐	☐	☐	☐	☐	☐	☐	☐
2	☐	☐	☐	☐	☐	☐	☐	☐	☐	☐
3	☐	☐	☐	☐	☐	☐	☐	☐	☐	☐
4	☐	☐	☐	☐	☐	☐	☐	☐	☐	☐
5	☐	☐	☐	☐	☐	☐	☐	☐	☐	☐

Period Symptoms

Discomfort: ☐ Cramps ☐ Mood Swings ☐ Headache ☐ Hunger
☐ Tender Breasts ☐ Back Pain ☐ Fatigue ☐ Acne ☐ Sleep Issues

Digestion: ☐ Nausea ☐ Ache ☐ Bloat ☐ Diarrhea ☐ Constipation

Cravings: ☐ Sweet ☐ Spice ☐ Salt ☐ Carb ☐ Cheese ☐ Alcohol

Emotions: ☐ Happy ☐ Energetic ☐ Motivated ☐ Calm ☐ Angry
☐ Irritated ☐ Sad ☐ Stressed ☐ Anxious ☐ Excited ☐ In Love

Body Check   *Weight:* _____

Exercise: ☐ Stretches ☐ Yoga ☐ Cardio ☐ Weights ☐ Impact

Diet: ☐ Healthy Eating ☐ Standard Diet ☐ Processed Food

Discharge Normal Colors: ☐ Clear ☐ White ☐ Pink ☐ Brown
  NOT Normal: ☐ Yellow ☐ Green ☐ Gray ☐ White Lumps

Problems: ☐ Itchy ☐ Burning ☐ Soreness ☐ Weird Discharge
☐ Funky Smell ☐ Odd Changes ☐ Pain with Peeing ☐ Pain with Sex

Sex: ☐ Nope ☐ Solo ☐ Girls Only ☐ Protected ☐ Unprotected

Birth Control: ☐ Condom ☐ IUD ☐ Pill ☐ Patch ☐ Implant
☐ Shot ☐ Vaginal Ring ☐ Tubal Ligation ☐ Partner Vasectomy

Notes

_____

_____

_____

_____

_____

_____

My Period   *Month:_____   Year:_____*

Start	SUN	MON	TUE	WED	THU	FRI	SAT
End							
Day Length							
Next Period Expected							

Arrived:

☐ On Time ☐ Early ☐ Late

Feels:

☐ Normal ☐ See Doc

FLOW	1	2	3	4	5	6	7	8	9	10
Spotting	☐	☐	☐	☐	☐	☐	☐	☐	☐	☐
Light	☐	☐	☐	☐	☐	☐	☐	☐	☐	☐
Medium	☐	☐	☐	☐	☐	☐	☐	☐	☐	☐
Heavy	☐	☐	☐	☐	☐	☐	☐	☐	☐	☐
Ultra	☐	☐	☐	☐	☐	☐	☐	☐	☐	☐
PAIN 1	☐	☐	☐	☐	☐	☐	☐	☐	☐	☐
2	☐	☐	☐	☐	☐	☐	☐	☐	☐	☐
3	☐	☐	☐	☐	☐	☐	☐	☐	☐	☐
4	☐	☐	☐	☐	☐	☐	☐	☐	☐	☐
5	☐	☐	☐	☐	☐	☐	☐	☐	☐	☐

Period Symptoms

Discomfort: ☐ Cramps ☐ Mood Swings ☐ Headache ☐ Hunger
☐ Tender Breasts ☐ Back Pain ☐ Fatigue ☐ Acne ☐ Sleep Issues

Digestion: ☐ Nausea ☐ Ache ☐ Bloat ☐ Diarrhea ☐ Constipation

Cravings: ☐ Sweet ☐ Spice ☐ Salt ☐ Carb ☐ Cheese ☐ Alcohol

Emotions: ☐ Happy ☐ Energetic ☐ Motivated ☐ Calm ☐ Angry
☐ Irritated ☐ Sad ☐ Stressed ☐ Anxious ☐ Excited ☐ In Love

Body Check   *Weight:* _____

Exercise: ☐ Stretches ☐ Yoga ☐ Cardio ☐ Weights ☐ Impact

Diet: ☐ Healthy Eating ☐ Standard Diet ☐ Processed Food

Discharge Normal Colors: ☐ Clear ☐ White ☐ Pink ☐ Brown
NOT Normal: ☐ Yellow ☐ Green ☐ Gray ☐ White Lumps

Problems: ☐ Itchy ☐ Burning ☐ Soreness ☐ Weird Discharge
☐ Funky Smell ☐ Odd Changes ☐ Pain with Peeing ☐ Pain with Sex

Sex: ☐ Nope ☐ Solo ☐ Girls Only ☐ Protected ☐ Unprotected

Birth Control: ☐ Condom ☐ IUD ☐ Pill ☐ Patch ☐ Implant
☐ Shot ☐ Vaginal Ring ☐ Tubal Ligation ☐ Partner Vasectomy

Notes

_____

_____

_____

_____

_____

_____

My Period　　*Month:*_____　*Year:*_____

Start	SUN	MON	TUE	WED	THU	FRI	SAT

End

Day Length

Next Period Expected

Arrived:

☐ On Time ☐ Early ☐ Late

Feels:

☐ Normal ☐ See Doc

FLOW	1	2	3	4	5	6	7	8	9	10
Spotting	☐	☐	☐	☐	☐	☐	☐	☐	☐	☐
Light	☐	☐	☐	☐	☐	☐	☐	☐	☐	☐
Medium	☐	☐	☐	☐	☐	☐	☐	☐	☐	☐
Heavy	☐	☐	☐	☐	☐	☐	☐	☐	☐	☐
Ultra	☐	☐	☐	☐	☐	☐	☐	☐	☐	☐
PAIN 1	☐	☐	☐	☐	☐	☐	☐	☐	☐	☐
2	☐	☐	☐	☐	☐	☐	☐	☐	☐	☐
3	☐	☐	☐	☐	☐	☐	☐	☐	☐	☐
4	☐	☐	☐	☐	☐	☐	☐	☐	☐	☐
5	☐	☐	☐	☐	☐	☐	☐	☐	☐	☐

Period Symptoms

Discomfort: ☐ Cramps ☐ Mood Swings ☐ Headache ☐ Hunger
☐ Tender Breasts ☐ Back Pain ☐ Fatigue ☐ Acne ☐ Sleep Issues

Digestion: ☐ Nausea ☐ Ache ☐ Bloat ☐ Diarrhea ☐ Constipation

Cravings: ☐ Sweet ☐ Spice ☐ Salt ☐ Carb ☐ Cheese ☐ Alcohol

Emotions: ☐ Happy ☐ Energetic ☐ Motivated ☐ Calm ☐ Angry
☐ Irritated ☐ Sad ☐ Stressed ☐ Anxious ☐ Excited ☐ In Love

Body Check   Weight: _____

Exercise: ☐ Stretches ☐ Yoga ☐ Cardio ☐ Weights ☐ Impact

Diet: ☐ Healthy Eating ☐ Standard Diet ☐ Processed Food

Discharge Normal Colors: ☐ Clear ☐ White ☐ Pink ☐ Brown
NOT Normal: ☐ Yellow ☐ Green ☐ Gray ☐ White Lumps

Problems: ☐ Itchy ☐ Burning ☐ Soreness ☐ Weird Discharge
☐ Funky Smell ☐ Odd Changes ☐ Pain with Peeing ☐ Pain with Sex

Sex: ☐ Nope ☐ Solo ☐ Girls Only ☐ Protected ☐ Unprotected

Birth Control: ☐ Condom ☐ IUD ☐ Pill ☐ Patch ☐ Implant
☐ Shot ☐ Vaginal Ring ☐ Tubal Ligation ☐ Partner Vasectomy

Notes

_____

_____

_____

_____

_____

_____

My Period   *Month:*_____   *Year:*_____

Start	SUN	MON	TUE	WED	THU	FRI	SAT
End							
Day Length							
Next Period Expected							

Arrived:

☐ On Time   ☐ Early   ☐ Late

Feels:

☐ Normal   ☐ See Doc

FLOW	1	2	3	4	5	6	7	8	9	10
Spotting	☐	☐	☐	☐	☐	☐	☐	☐	☐	☐
Light	☐	☐	☐	☐	☐	☐	☐	☐	☐	☐
Medium	☐	☐	☐	☐	☐	☐	☐	☐	☐	☐
Heavy	☐	☐	☐	☐	☐	☐	☐	☐	☐	☐
Ultra	☐	☐	☐	☐	☐	☐	☐	☐	☐	☐
PAIN 1	☐	☐	☐	☐	☐	☐	☐	☐	☐	☐
2	☐	☐	☐	☐	☐	☐	☐	☐	☐	☐
3	☐	☐	☐	☐	☐	☐	☐	☐	☐	☐
4	☐	☐	☐	☐	☐	☐	☐	☐	☐	☐
5	☐	☐	☐	☐	☐	☐	☐	☐	☐	☐

Period Symptoms

Discomfort: ☐ Cramps ☐ Mood Swings ☐ Headache ☐ Hunger ☐ Tender Breasts ☐ Back Pain ☐ Fatigue ☐ Acne ☐ Sleep Issues

Digestion: ☐ Nausea ☐ Ache ☐ Bloat ☐ Diarrhea ☐ Constipation

Cravings: ☐ Sweet ☐ Spice ☐ Salt ☐ Carb ☐ Cheese ☐ Alcohol

Emotions: ☐ Happy ☐ Energetic ☐ Motivated ☐ Calm ☐ Angry ☐ Irritated ☐ Sad ☐ Stressed ☐ Anxious ☐ Excited ☐ In Love

Body Check   *Weight:* _____

Exercise: ☐ Stretches ☐ Yoga ☐ Cardio ☐ Weights ☐ Impact

Diet: ☐ Healthy Eating ☐ Standard Diet ☐ Processed Food

Discharge Normal Colors: ☐ Clear ☐ White ☐ Pink ☐ Brown **NOT Normal:** ☐ Yellow ☐ Green ☐ Gray ☐ White Lumps

Problems: ☐ Itchy ☐ Burning ☐ Soreness ☐ Weird Discharge ☐ Funky Smell ☐ Odd Changes ☐ Pain with Peeing ☐ Pain with Sex

Sex: ☐ Nope ☐ Solo ☐ Girls Only ☐ Protected ☐ Unprotected

Birth Control: ☐ Condom ☐ IUD ☐ Pill ☐ Patch ☐ Implant ☐ Shot ☐ Vaginal Ring ☐ Tubal Ligation ☐ Partner Vasectomy

Notes

_____

_____

_____

_____

_____

_____

My Period   *Month:_____   Year:_____*

Start	SUN	MON	TUE	WED	THU	FRI	SAT
End							
Day Length							
Next Period Expected							

Arrived:

☐ On Time ☐ Early ☐ Late

Feels:

☐ Normal ☐ See Doc

FLOW	1	2	3	4	5	6	7	8	9	10
Spotting	☐	☐	☐	☐	☐	☐	☐	☐	☐	☐
Light	☐	☐	☐	☐	☐	☐	☐	☐	☐	☐
Medium	☐	☐	☐	☐	☐	☐	☐	☐	☐	☐
Heavy	☐	☐	☐	☐	☐	☐	☐	☐	☐	☐
Ultra	☐	☐	☐	☐	☐	☐	☐	☐	☐	☐
PAIN 1	☐	☐	☐	☐	☐	☐	☐	☐	☐	☐
2	☐	☐	☐	☐	☐	☐	☐	☐	☐	☐
3	☐	☐	☐	☐	☐	☐	☐	☐	☐	☐
4	☐	☐	☐	☐	☐	☐	☐	☐	☐	☐
5	☐	☐	☐	☐	☐	☐	☐	☐	☐	☐

Period Symptoms

Discomfort: ☐ Cramps ☐ Mood Swings ☐ Headache ☐ Hunger
☐ Tender Breasts ☐ Back Pain ☐ Fatigue ☐ Acne ☐ Sleep Issues

Digestion: ☐ Nausea ☐ Ache ☐ Bloat ☐ Diarrhea ☐ Constipation

Cravings: ☐ Sweet ☐ Spice ☐ Salt ☐ Carb ☐ Cheese ☐ Alcohol

Emotions: ☐ Happy ☐ Energetic ☐ Motivated ☐ Calm ☐ Angry
☐ Irritated ☐ Sad ☐ Stressed ☐ Anxious ☐ Excited ☐ In Love

Body Check   *Weight:* _____

Exercise: ☐ Stretches ☐ Yoga ☐ Cardio ☐ Weights ☐ Impact

Diet: ☐ Healthy Eating ☐ Standard Diet ☐ Processed Food

Discharge Normal Colors: ☐ Clear ☐ White ☐ Pink ☐ Brown
  NOT Normal: ☐ Yellow ☐ Green ☐ Gray ☐ White Lumps

Problems: ☐ Itchy ☐ Burning ☐ Soreness ☐ Weird Discharge
☐ Funky Smell ☐ Odd Changes ☐ Pain with Peeing ☐ Pain with Sex

Sex: ☐ Nope ☐ Solo ☐ Girls Only ☐ Protected ☐ Unprotected

Birth Control: ☐ Condom ☐ IUD ☐ Pill ☐ Patch ☐ Implant
☐ Shot ☐ Vaginal Ring ☐ Tubal Ligation ☐ Partner Vasectomy

Notes

_____

_____

_____

_____

_____

_____

My Period   *Month:*_____   *Year:*_____

	SUN	MON	TUE	WED	THU	FRI	SAT
Start							
End							
Day Length							
Next Period Expected							

Arrived:

☐ On Time ☐ Early ☐ Late

Feels:

☐ Normal ☐ See Doc

FLOW	1	2	3	4	5	6	7	8	9	10
Spotting	☐	☐	☐	☐	☐	☐	☐	☐	☐	☐
Light	☐	☐	☐	☐	☐	☐	☐	☐	☐	☐
Medium	☐	☐	☐	☐	☐	☐	☐	☐	☐	☐
Heavy	☐	☐	☐	☐	☐	☐	☐	☐	☐	☐
Ultra	☐	☐	☐	☐	☐	☐	☐	☐	☐	☐
PAIN 1	☐	☐	☐	☐	☐	☐	☐	☐	☐	☐
2	☐	☐	☐	☐	☐	☐	☐	☐	☐	☐
3	☐	☐	☐	☐	☐	☐	☐	☐	☐	☐
4	☐	☐	☐	☐	☐	☐	☐	☐	☐	☐
5	☐	☐	☐	☐	☐	☐	☐	☐	☐	☐

Period Symptoms

Discomfort: ☐ Cramps ☐ Mood Swings ☐ Headache ☐ Hunger ☐ Tender Breasts ☐ Back Pain ☐ Fatigue ☐ Acne ☐ Sleep Issues

Digestion: ☐ Nausea ☐ Ache ☐ Bloat ☐ Diarrhea ☐ Constipation

Cravings: ☐ Sweet ☐ Spice ☐ Salt ☐ Carb ☐ Cheese ☐ Alcohol

Emotions: ☐ Happy ☐ Energetic ☐ Motivated ☐ Calm ☐ Angry ☐ Irritated ☐ Sad ☐ Stressed ☐ Anxious ☐ Excited ☐ In Love

Body Check   *Weight:* _____

Exercise: ☐ Stretches ☐ Yoga ☐ Cardio ☐ Weights ☐ Impact

Diet: ☐ Healthy Eating ☐ Standard Diet ☐ Processed Food

Discharge Normal Colors: ☐ Clear ☐ White ☐ Pink ☐ Brown
NOT Normal: ☐ Yellow ☐ Green ☐ Gray ☐ White Lumps

Problems: ☐ Itchy ☐ Burning ☐ Soreness ☐ Weird Discharge ☐ Funky Smell ☐ Odd Changes ☐ Pain with Peeing ☐ Pain with Sex

Sex: ☐ Nope ☐ Solo ☐ Girls Only ☐ Protected ☐ Unprotected

Birth Control: ☐ Condom ☐ IUD ☐ Pill ☐ Patch ☐ Implant ☐ Shot ☐ Vaginal Ring ☐ Tubal Ligation ☐ Partner Vasectomy

Notes

_____

_____

_____

_____

_____

_____

My Period   Month:_____   Year:_____

Start

SUN	MON	TUE	WED	THU	FRI	SAT

End

Day Length

Next Period Expected

Arrived:

☐ On Time ☐ Early ☐ Late

Feels:

☐ Normal ☐ See Doc

FLOW	1	2	3	4	5	6	7	8	9	10
Spotting	☐	☐	☐	☐	☐	☐	☐	☐	☐	☐
Light	☐	☐	☐	☐	☐	☐	☐	☐	☐	☐
Medium	☐	☐	☐	☐	☐	☐	☐	☐	☐	☐
Heavy	☐	☐	☐	☐	☐	☐	☐	☐	☐	☐
Ultra	☐	☐	☐	☐	☐	☐	☐	☐	☐	☐
PAIN 1	☐	☐	☐	☐	☐	☐	☐	☐	☐	☐
2	☐	☐	☐	☐	☐	☐	☐	☐	☐	☐
3	☐	☐	☐	☐	☐	☐	☐	☐	☐	☐
4	☐	☐	☐	☐	☐	☐	☐	☐	☐	☐
5	☐	☐	☐	☐	☐	☐	☐	☐	☐	☐

Period Symptoms

Discomfort: ☐ Cramps ☐ Mood Swings ☐ Headache ☐ Hunger
☐ Tender Breasts ☐ Back Pain ☐ Fatigue ☐ Acne ☐ Sleep Issues

Digestion: ☐ Nausea ☐ Ache ☐ Bloat ☐ Diarrhea ☐ Constipation

Cravings: ☐ Sweet ☐ Spice ☐ Salt ☐ Carb ☐ Cheese ☐ Alcohol

Emotions: ☐ Happy ☐ Energetic ☐ Motivated ☐ Calm ☐ Angry
☐ Irritated ☐ Sad ☐ Stressed ☐ Anxious ☐ Excited ☐ In Love

Body Check   *Weight:* _____

Exercise: ☐ Stretches ☐ Yoga ☐ Cardio ☐ Weights ☐ Impact

Diet: ☐ Healthy Eating ☐ Standard Diet ☐ Processed Food

Discharge Normal Colors: ☐ Clear ☐ White ☐ Pink ☐ Brown
  NOT Normal: ☐ Yellow ☐ Green ☐ Gray ☐ White Lumps

Problems: ☐ Itchy ☐ Burning ☐ Soreness ☐ Weird Discharge
☐ Funky Smell ☐ Odd Changes ☐ Pain with Peeing ☐ Pain with Sex

Sex: ☐ Nope ☐ Solo ☐ Girls Only ☐ Protected ☐ Unprotected

Birth Control: ☐ Condom ☐ IUD ☐ Pill ☐ Patch ☐ Implant
☐ Shot ☐ Vaginal Ring ☐ Tubal Ligation ☐ Partner Vasectomy

Notes

_____

_____

_____

_____

_____

_____

	1	2	3	4	5	6	7	8	9	10	11	12	13	14	15	16	17	18	19	20	21	22	23	24	25	26	27	28	29	30	31
Jan																															
Feb																															
Mar																															
Apr																															
May																															
Jun																															
Jul																															
Aug																															
Sep																															
Oct																															
Nov																															
Dec																															

	1	2	3	4	5	6	7	8	9	10	11	12	13	14	15	16	17	18	19	20	21	22	23	24	25	26	27	28	29	30	31
Jan																															
Feb																															
Mar																															
Apr																															
May																															
Jun																															
Jul																															
Aug																															
Sep																															
Oct																															
Nov																															
Dec																															

	1	2	3	4	5	6	7	8	9	10	11	12	13	14	15	16	17	18	19	20	21	22	23	24	25	26	27	28	29	30	31
Jan																															
Feb																															
Mar																															
Apr																															
May																															
Jun																															
Jul																															
Aug																															
Sep																															
Oct																															
Nov																															
Dec																															

	1	2	3	4	5	6	7	8	9	10	11	12	13	14	15	16	17	18	19	20	21	22	23	24	25	26	27	28	29	30	31
Jan																															
Feb																															
Mar																															
Apr																															
May																															
Jun																															
Jul																															
Aug																															
Sep																															
Oct																															
Nov																															
Dec																															

	1	2	3	4	5	6	7	8	9	10	11	12	13	14	15	16	17	18	19	20	21	22	23	24	25	26	27	28	29	30	31
Jan																															
Feb																															
Mar																															
Apr																															
May																															
Jun																															
Jul																															
Aug																															
Sep																															
Oct																															
Nov																															
Dec																															

Made in the USA
Columbia, SC
18 March 2025

55363121R00072